## Praise for the bestselling *Fast Diet*:

'The biggest diet revolution since the Atkins.'
*Daily Mail*

'I think I might just be part of a health revolution.'
*Hugh Fearnley-Whittingstall*

'The Fast Diet is ideal for those of us who
can just about manage to be good, but lack the
long distance rigour of saints.'
*Allison Pearson*

'The TV diet that works.'
*Radio Times*

'Amazing... The only diet you'll ever need.'
*Mail on Sunday*

'Fasting two days in seven isn't so hard, unlike the
diets that need steely resolve 24/7.'
*Daily Express*

'2013's hottest regime.'
*Grazia*

# fast
## exercise

# fast
## exercise

# DR MICHAEL MOSLEY

## WITH PETA BEE

Foreword by Professor Jamie Timmons
Loughborough University

The information contained in this book is provided for general purposes only. It is not intended as and should not be relied upon as medical advice. The publisher and authors are not responsible for any specific health needs that may require medical supervision. If you have underlying health problems, or have any doubts about the advice contained in this book, you should contact a qualified medical, dietary, or other appropriate professional.

Published in 2013 by Short Books
Unit 316, ScreenWorks
22 Highbury Grove
London N5 2ER

17

A CIP catalogue record for this book is available from the British Library.
ISBN 978-1-78072-198-9

Printed in Great Britain by CPI Group (UK) Ltd. Croydon, CR0 4YY

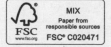

MIX
Paper from
responsible sources
FSC® C020471

For Clare, Alex, Jack, Daniel and Kate –
who I want to stay fit and strong for.

# CONTENTS

# FOREWORD

Over the last couple of years I've noted a remarkable transformation in Dr Michael Mosley. Gone is the middle-aged spread I saw when we first met and in its place are super-efficient muscles, doing a good job of rapidly clearing away the high levels of sugar and fat that used to hang around in his arteries after each meal. I flatter myself that at least part of this transformation stems from our work together, in 2011, on a documentary – for which we put Michael through his paces in our lab and introduced him to high intensity training (or HIT for short).

Michael was at that time searching for solutions to combat his family history of Type 2 diabetes – solutions which he knew would include exercise, but ideally in a form that was as brief and effective as possible. The reason we met was because my team in Edinburgh had recently completed a study, demonstrating that just a few minutes of high intensity cycling a week could dramatically improve your diabetes risk factors.

This sounds, on the surface, like an absurd claim. We 'know' that to get the benefits of exercise, like aerobic and metabolic fitness, you have to put in the hours. But is that really true?

When I was 12 years old I ran my first half-marathon in Renfrew, Scotland. Over the following 10 years I must have run over 20,000 miles, and also completed many hours of gym training. I did so because this is what science told us was required to improve aerobic performance.

Even before starting at Glasgow University (to become a dentist, of all things), I was an avid reader of exercise science books. During my intercalated degree studies, which focused on exercise physiology, I began to realise that much of the classic exercise science – carried out only by athletes or small numbers of super-healthy Scandinavians – was not a reliable guide to how exercise modifies health and physiology in the general public.

My first introduction to HIT was not, however, in a lecture theatre but on the track. Early in the track season my coach, John Toner, had me doing sets of 3 x 200m with 3 minutes of recovery and not much more. This was not normal training for a distance runner, but it at least had the virtue of being quick. I was intrigued.

During my last year at Glasgow, I decided to carry out a training intervention study as my honours project. Working with the youth team at our athletics club, we put them through 10 weeks of high intensity interval training and found improvements in performance and efficiency way beyond what was achieved through regular endurance training. Just after graduating, I presented my findings at my first scientific conference, organised by McMaster University, fittingly enough where modern 'cycle-based' HIT was born.

Since then I have spent 20 years working on human physiology, exercise and genomics, trying to explain the links between exercise and health. For the past 10 years, at our university laboratories in the UK, in Scandinavia and with colleagues in Canada, we have put hundreds of volunteers through different forms of HIT. Medical tests have shown that just a few minutes of HIT, done 3 times a week, can deliver improvements in line with the benefits you'd get from doing many hours of conventional exercise.

Importantly, these findings have come out of independent studies done in several countries – notably by professors Martin Gibala at McMaster University in Canada, Niels Vollaard at the University of Bath and Ulrik Wisloff in Norway.

One of the reasons we do this research is because we are interested in time. Or rather the lack of it. We all know there are good reasons for doing exercise. As well as improving fitness, there are long-term health benefits in reducing risk factors associated with cancer, diabetes and cardiovascular disease.

But we also know that following conventional exercise recommendations involves time and effort. Critically lack of time is the most common reason people give for not doing any organised physical activity.

I believe that we have now produced sufficient data to be able to recommend short bursts of high intensity exercise as a safe and effective alternative to conventional workouts, removing the 'time barrier' as an excuse for not exercising. This will hopefully boost compliance and help people to take up an approach that will lead to a healthier way of life. The great thing about HIT is that it can be done in the workplace or at home without pre-planning or missing an episode of your favourite TV show.

I also believe that when it comes to advances in exercise science, we have only begun to scratch the surface, that our increased understanding of genomics and metabolomics will soon help us tailor or personalise life-style advice.

Once upon a time we assumed that everyone got roughly the same benefit from exercise and that if people didn't it was because they were slacking. Today we know that the way each person responds to exercise is unique and we can use genomic testing to help personalise goal setting.

By early 2013 nearly a million people in the USA had already signed up for full genome-scans with the hope of understanding their health better and avoiding the risk factors most relevant to their genes. Tailored advice is better advice and better advice should reduce chronic disease, ultimately reducing pressure on our public health services. By combining simple solutions like HIT with hi-tech solutions like DNA profiling we hope to pinpoint the optimal exercise protocol to help control the risk factors most relevant to each individual and not some abstract population 'average'.

Doing the science is critical. But without translation of this 'science' into a useful and practical guide, one that can be used by anyone, our science fails to make an impact.

I recommend *Fast Exercise* because it is an up-to-date account of the latest studies but one which also demystifies some quite complex science, opening eyes to how easily an exercise regime can fit into a daily routine.

Following Michael and Peta's advice, and our science, should help you reduce your risk of various chronic diseases and, who knows, you may even find yourself enjoying a workout for the first time!

*Professor Jamie Timmons PhD, UK*
*December 2013*

# INTRODUCTION

As a medically trained journalist I frequently come across claims that seem too good to be true and often are. Occasionally, after digging around, I reconsider my original position, acknowledge that what might appear at first to be outrageous could have something in it. As the economist John Maynard Keynes once said, 'When the facts change, I change my mind.'

This happened to me when, in early 2012, I first heard about intermittent fasting. My initial reaction was scepticism. I assumed it would turn out to be some variation on 'detoxing' or other largely discredited views of how the body works. Nonetheless I decided to find out more as I'd recently discovered that I was a borderline diabetic with too much visceral fat (the fat that lies inside your abdomen). My father had died from a diabetes-related illness and I could see myself going down the same road.

So I set out to examine the claim that you can lose weight and get health benefits, particularly improvements in your insulin, by changing your pattern of eating. I soon came across research done in the US and the UK which pointed to rapid fat loss and other benefits that would come from cutting my calories, not every day, but just a few days a week.

As I looked deeper I discovered intermittent fasting was backed by a significant body of animal and human research. I spoke to many eminent experts, tested the claims on myself, and made a documentary for the BBC. Then, in January 2013, I wrote a book with Mimi Spencer, *The Fast Diet*, which summarised all this research into what we called a 5:2 diet (eat normally 5 days a week, cut your calories for 2). Using this method, I lost over 20lb of fat and my blood glucose returned to a normal level. Although this was just my experience (and personal anecdotes make poor science) it was in line with a number of clinical studies done on different forms of intermittent fasting.

We still don't know the ideal pattern for intermittent fasting, the true long-term benefits or the potential pitfalls, but since the book was published many thousands of people have followed the 5:2 regime, lost weight and contacted me to say how easy it is. And I'm pleased to say new studies are underway.

While writing *The Fast Diet*, one of the areas I touched on – but only briefly – was exercise. Diet and exercise are complementary, they go together like Fred Astaire and Ginger Rogers, like Batman and Robin. And, as we will see, there are interesting parallels in the way science is transforming the way we think about both.

Before making the film on fasting, I had come across a rapidly developing new area of exercise research called High Intensity Interval Training (HIIT), also known as HIT (High Intensity Training).

One of the pioneers of this radically different approach to exercise is Jamie Timmons, Professor of Systems Biology at Loughborough University. Loughborough is home to the Centre for Olympic Studies and Research and has one of the leading sports research departments in the UK.

When we met, Jamie made what I thought was an outrageous, almost unbelievable claim. He said that I could get many of the more important benefits of exercise from just 3 minutes of intense exercise a week. He said that if I was prepared to give it a go he was confident that in just 4 weeks I would see significant changes in my biochemistry. It seemed wildly unlikely but also immensely intriguing. So I got myself properly tested and then I went for it. The results, which I discuss on page 81, were a revelation.

Since I had an initial conversation with Jamie back in 2011, research on HIT has exploded, with new findings coming out all the time. Even in the 18 months that I have been working on this book there has been a wealth of new studies providing mounting evidence that you really can get many of the same benefits, from short bursts of intense effort as you can from following the more traditional approach, or perhaps even more. Benefits which include:

- Improved aerobic fitness and endurance

- Reduced body fat

- Increased upper and lower body strength

- Improved insulin sensitivity

These research findings form the basis of what I've called Fast Exercise, a practical and enjoyable way to get the maximal benefits in the minimal time.

My co-author, leading sports journalist and coach Peta Bee, has spent her career investigating the claims of the sport and fitness industry. Unlike me she loves exercise. She's provided invaluable experience which has helped turn theory into practice.

## The Dynamo & the Slob

### Michael's motivation

Peta and I approach exercise from very different perspectives. She is fantastically sporty and has been from an early age. She runs marathons for fun and adores a good hard workout. She has spent the last 20 years thinking, writing and training others to share her passion.

I, on the other hand, don't like exercise. I don't get a high from working out or pushing myself; instead I share the views of astronaut Neil Armstrong who once said, 'I believe that every human has a finite amount of heartbeats. I don't intend to waste any of mine running around doing exercises.' Or the actor Peter O'Toole who claimed, 'The only exercise I take is walking behind the coffins of friends who took exercise.'

All right, that is an exaggeration. Now aged 56, I see the need and I appreciate the value of being active. I also fully embrace the idea that we are born to move. When I was at medical school I played quite a lot of sport, went for runs and swam. Then I started working and could no longer find the time.

Don't get me wrong; I am not a complete slob. I love skiing, enjoy walks, relish swimming in the sea and like being active. I don't actually think of any of these as 'exercise', something you do because you think you should.

Exercise for me means the gym. It means going for long runs even when it is wet and cold, or trudging away on the treadmill; it is hours getting sweaty on an exercise bike or lifting heavy weights, followed by those incredulous moments when you step on the weighing scales and discover that you have hardly shifted a pound. For me, exercise is there to be endured, done because you have to, not because you want to.

If I am going to exercise I want it to be short, sharp, easy to do and soon over. This, along with the science, is what first attracted me to HIT. Peta, as you might expect, came to HIT for different reasons.

## Peta's motivation

Unlike Michael, I love exercise and the way it makes me feel. I enjoy testing my own endurance and strength and relish the fatigue that comes with being absolutely physically spent.

My love affair with exercise started when I took up athletics at primary school – a start which eventually saw me run for Wales in my teens and early twenties. My passion for understanding how the body responds to intense effort, how it is repeatedly able to push itself to new limits, led me to study sports science at university. It was during that time that I gained a grounding in the basic principles of physiology and biomechanics and this cemented my view of fitness and how to attain it. Fitness eventually became the prime focus of my career as a journalist, and for the past 20 years I have written about sports science and fitness and their impact on health and longevity.

As for HIT, in all my many years of exercising and studying the practice of exercise, I have found nothing that comes close to producing the physical and mental rewards of it. I suppose in some ways I am the living embodiment of a lifelong Fast Exerciser – not that I realised it until recently. My induction into the concept of intense bursts of effort with short bouts of recovery occurred when I first started athletics training. Several times a week I would sprint-jog, sprint-jog my way around the track – a practice I have kept up with varying degrees of effort to this day as I race up hills, around alternate edges of a football pitch, between lampposts and along lines of trees.

Now, at 45, a busy, working mum, I no longer have the time or, to be honest, the inclination to spend more than an hour a day working out. Yes, I want to offset middle-age weight gain, to feel good and, of course, look as good as I can. And I want a body that performs well. But I want it fast. And that, in short, is the greatest appeal of HIT for me. If you want to discover a way to get fit quickly, with minimal time commitment, read on.

The role of science is to question. It is by doing experiments that traditional thinking is challenged and sometimes overthrown. So, where does that leave widely held exercise beliefs? Claims such as:

- To get maximum benefit you should do lots of moderate intensity exercise

- If you exercise you will lose weight

- You should always do lengthy warm-ups before exercising

- Stretching before exercise will improve your performance and reduce your risk of injury

- We all get benefit from doing exercise

In this book we take a good, hard look at these and other claims. In the first part, Michael looks at the history and science of HIT, and his own attempts to put theory into practice. In the second part, Peta has put together a range of evidence-based Fast Exercise workouts, along with practical advice and tips on how to integrate HIT into your life.

We want you to be as sceptical about our conclusions as we are about others'. We have included numerous references to the scientific literature that we have drawn on so that you can make your own judgments. These studies can be easily accessed through an internet search; most are free in their entirety; all are available as abstracts.

We owe an enormous debt of gratitude to the numerous scientists and volunteers who have devoted their time and their bodies to uncovering the truths about exercise and who have put themselves through a range of strenuous routines in the hope of discovering the optimal ways to work out.

No one size will fit all but we hope this book will give you the information you need to create an effective and enjoyable exercise regime that works for you.

This is a book for those who, like Michael, don't enjoy exercise but who want to keep down the fat and stay healthy in the most effective, time-efficient way. It is for those, like Peta, who love exercise and want to get the most from it. It is also for those who are simply curious about themselves and who like having their preconceptions challenged. Enjoy.

# THE TRUTH ABOUT
# EXERCISE

Even on a day when it's cold and grey outside and the last thing you want to do is pull on your trainers, there are good reasons for getting up and going out. Regular exercise is a powerful anti-aging medicine, providing a wide range of health and psychological benefits, from strengthening your bones to improving your brain, from reducing cancer risk to boosting your mood. You might even look better on the beach.

Yet exercise, like diet, is an area that is swathed in popular misconceptions. There is a huge gap between what sports scientists know about exercise and what is actually done in gyms and public parks. In recent years new studies have overturned much of what we once thought was well established.

Based on the latest research, this book will reveal, among other things:

- How to get fit in a few minutes a day

- Why some people get so much more benefit from exercise than others

- Why high-volume, low intensity exercise like jogging rarely leads to weight loss

This last claim is in many ways the most surprising and disheartening. After all, the main reason why many of us take up jogging or join a gym is because we believe it will help us shed the pounds. Burn calories, lose weight.

If only things were so simple. Study after study has shown that conventional, low intensity exercise like jogging or swimming rarely leads to weight loss. If you want to lose fat then intensity is the key.

## So what are the measurable benefits of exercise?

### *Exercise and longevity*

One of the things we'd all expect regular exercise would lead to is a longer, healthier life. But how active do you need to be and what sort of exercise should you be doing?

Thanks to a recent review of 22 separate studies[1] which followed nearly a million people from Europe, North

America, East Asia and Australasia, we know that a couch potato who gets off the sofa and starts doing around 2.5 hours of moderate activity a week (walking, cycling, jogging, swimming) can expect to reduce their mortality risk by around 19%.

That sounds pretty impressive and it is the sort of figure bandied around by experts in the hope that it will encourage people to move more. The trouble is, it doesn't. Despite numerous public health campaigns, most Europeans and North Americans don't come close to doing 2.5 hours of moderate activity a week. Fewer than 20% of us do anything like the recommended levels.

There are many barriers to getting more active (lack of time is the commonest excuse), but I also think the way in which the benefits of exercise are presented is not particularly compelling or convincing.

'Mortality risk', for example, is a concept that is difficult to grasp and not a great motivator. To get a better grip on what 'mortality risk' means I asked a statistician friend to try and explain this finding in a more comprehensible way.

After grinding the numbers he concluded that if you are bone idle and start doing about 20 minutes of exercise a day then that will add about 2.2 years to your life expectancy.

Adding 2.2 years to life expectancy sounds reasonable, but if to get this return I have to exercise 2.5 hours a week and I don't particularly enjoy it, is that really a good investment of my time? And if I do more will I get more benefit?

Fortunately, there is another, more interesting way of looking at this sort of data. It is called 'Microlives', and it is the brainchild of Professor David Spiegelhalter of Cambridge University. It is a brave attempt to turn complex studies into understandable facts.

What Professor Spiegelhalter realised is that once you hit your mid-twenties you can expect to live around 57 more years. Fifty seven years conveniently translates into half a million hours, or a million 30-minute chunks of life. These 30-minute chunks he calls microlives.

Based on this idea, Professor Spiegelhalter went through lots of studies[2] and started calculating the number of microlives you win or lose by doing a range of different activities. Smoking 20 cigarettes a day, for example, shortens your life expectancy by around 8 years. This means that every pack of cigarettes you smoke will reduce your life by around 10 microlives or about 5 hours.

On the other hand, each portion of fruit and vegetables you eat adds just under 1 microlife, so if you eat the recommended 5 portions a day you should get an extra 4 years of life, mainly because of your reduced risk of heart disease.

I was pleased to see that, according to the *New England Journal of Medicine*, drinking a moderate amount of coffee is good for you. In fact, it turns out that drinking 2-3 cups of coffee a day (and it doesn't seem to matter much whether it is caffeinated or not) will add 1 microlife – possibly thanks to the flavonoids in it which have an antioxidant effect. This means that the 2 cups of coffee I drink every morning not only make me sharper and cheerier afterwards, they are time well spent.

If I spend 10 minutes drinking coffee and each time I have a cup I am adding around 30 minutes to my life, then that looks like a real bargain. (Unfortunately, if you go much beyond 3 cups a day the benefits begin to fade.)

So how well does exercise compare with drinking coffee or eating vegetables? Pretty well, at least to start with. If you are a slob and start exercising for 20 minutes a day that will buy you 2 microlives – an extra hour of life.

But the benefits of doing more exercise, at least in terms of life expectancy, then drop off dramatically. This is not a linear relationship. If you decide to exercise for an hour a day this will not add 6 microlives. The extra 40 minutes of exercise will, at most, only get you 1 extra microlife.

In other words, after the first 20 minutes, the next 20 minutes of moderate exercise you do will only buy you an extra 15 minutes of life. If, like me, you don't enjoy those 20 minutes it begins to look like a rather bad investment.

This is all a bit artificial because there are clearly costs and benefits to be had that are not reflected in mortality statistics. If I smoke 20 cigarettes a day, for example, I am not only going to die younger, I am probably going to spend the last few decades of my life coughing, wheezing and generally feeling wretched. Similarly, if I exercise regularly I am likely to be more active, alert and taking fewer drugs in old age. In truth, most of us know which we would prefer.

## How exercise benefits your brain

I am very fond of my brain so I was particularly encouraged when I came across a number of studies that point out how good exercise is, not just for the body, but also for the brain.

In a study done at the University of Illinois,[3] they took 59 healthy but sedentary volunteers, aged 60-79, and randomly allocated them to one of two programmes: either aerobic training or 'toning and stretching' exercises done for 6 months. Before and after the volunteers did these exercises, they had scans to measure the size of their brains.

The results were extremely interesting: there were significant increases in the brain volume of those doing the fitness training, but not of those who just did the stretching and toning.

One reason why this happens may be because exercise leads to the release of all sorts of proteins in the brain, including BDNF (brain-derived neurotrophic factor). This protein helps protect existing brain cells and encourages the development of new ones.

So you get a bigger brain, but also one that is probably better protected against dementia.

In another intriguing study,[4] researchers followed 20,000 men and women who had had their baseline fitness measured between 1971 and 2009. During that time, 1,659 of them developed dementia. Scarily, the ones who were the least fit were almost twice as likely to succumb to dementia as those who were most fit.

This was not an exercise intervention study, so we do not know if embarking on a fitness programme will actually make a difference. But it seems plausible.

## So much for the benefits. What are the risks?

The evidence is strong that moving is much better than not moving; and, if you are like Peta and enjoy exercise for its own sake, then working out is time well spent, whatever the tangible health benefits. However, it is worth pointing out that recent studies suggest that more is not necessarily better.

We know, for example, that excessive exercise can lead to long-term damage of your joints.

My father, who was a keen rugby player when he was young, spent the last decade of his life in a lot of pain in his knees as a result of injuries which occurred when he was in his twenties. We know that arthritis of the lower joints (particularly knees) is far more common in footballers and some athletes than in the normal population, and a study of former PE teachers in Sweden turned up some pretty disturbing findings.

In a study published in the *Journal of Occupational and Environmental Health*,[5] researchers tracked down more than 500 men and women who had qualified from the Gymnastiska Centralinstitutet, a training college for PE teachers in Sweden, between 1957 and 1965. The subjects were, at the time of the study, mainly in their late fifties. The researchers then chose a matched group of people from the general Swedish population and did a comparison.

What they found was that the former PE teachers had far higher rates of arthritis of the knee and hip than the matched group of contemporaries. Despite being slimmer and more health-conscious, they were 3 times more likely to have arthritis in the knees than people from the general population. In fact, their problems were so severe that only 20% were still working as PE teachers, and in a number of cases their joints had needed replacement surgery.

Joint problems are common in impact sports, but oddly enough this is not the case among runners. If anything, running seems to be protective. The risk to runners who overdo it seems to be more from damage to the heart than to the joints.

An editorial, published in the June 2013 edition of the

*Journal of Applied Physiology*,[6] pointed out that half of serious rowers and marathon runners showed early signs of fibrosis in their hearts. Fibrosis, a form of scarring, can lead to irregular heartbeats which in turn can lead to more significant problems.

Before you get too worried I should stress that the men who were studied had undergone immense amounts of training, far more than the average distance runner, and this damage may be reversible, at least it is in rats.

Nonetheless, some cardiologists who study the impact of exercise are concerned about the effects of extreme endurance sports on the heart. The authors of this review (who were both once keen long-distance runners) point out that the very first marathon runner, Phidippides, a courier who ran the 26 miles from Marathon to Athens to announce news of a Greek victory, dropped dead on arrival.

The odds of that happening to a modern-day marathon runner are small, but as these cardiologists point out, 'chronic extreme exercise seems to cause wear and tear on the heart'.

Research from Denmark has also raised a few alarms about jogging too far and too fast.[7]

In 1975 a team in Copenhagen began following a group of 20,000 Danes aged between 20 and 93. Some did regular exercise, most did not. At the start of the study and throughout the years that followed, the volunteers kept a record of how much jogging they did, how far and how intensely. Over the course of the last 37 years more than 10,000 of the people in the study have died.

By comparing death rates between joggers and non-joggers, the researchers were able to show that jogging can add around 4 years to your life, which is in line with studies I mentioned earlier. This finding, when it was published, was widely reported. What was less covered was the finding that you seem to get the maximum benefits if you don't do too much.

The ideal, at least based on this study, is to jog for 30-50 minutes, 3 days a week, at a pace at which you feel 'a little breathless but not very breathless'. You can still chat but probably not sing. Recovery days are important, which is why it is better to jog 3 times a week than 20 minutes every day.

The sting in the tail is that beyond a certain point doing more exercise may be counter-productive. When the researchers looked at the data in detail they concluded that 'these results showed a tendency of a U-shaped relation to mortality risk'. In other words, doing some running is better than sitting on the sofa, but doing lots of running may not be better than doing a moderate amount.

We don't know at what point 'a lot' becomes 'too much' but if you are exercising for more than an hour a day you are probably doing it for reasons other than optimising your health.

## How can you tell if exercise is doing you any good?

It's all very well having big studies showing the average improvements in mortality that can be expected from doing different levels of exercise but most of us want advice that is more personal.

How do you know if a new exercise regime is improving *your* health, extending *your* life? The obvious measure, standing on the weighing scales, is not going to be particularly revealing – not only because the scales are unlikely to move much but because changes in weight are not the best predictor of future benefits (see page 50).

So what are the changes that matter? Increased strength and flexibility are important and we include a list at the back of the book of the sort of things you might want to measure before starting an exercise regime, but 2 of the most important measures are aerobic fitness and glucose tolerance.

### Aerobic fitness

Aerobic fitness refers to your endurance or ability to keep going while doing something like jogging or running. It is a measure of how strong your heart and lungs are and how well they respond to the stresses placed upon them.

The most widely accepted way of measuring aerobic fitness is VO2 max. This is the maximum amount of oxygen that your body can use while you are doing intense exercise. Another way of looking at it is that VO2 max is a measure of how good your heart and lungs are at getting oxygen into and round your body – how strong your engine is.

VO2 max is not just a measure of how fit you are, but a powerful predictor of future health. We worry about cholesterol, alcohol, being overweight. Yet none of these matter anything like as much as your VO2 max. People with good levels of aerobic fitness are much less likely to get heart disease, cancer, diabetes or become demented.

As we'll see in later chapters, most people's VO2 max rises quite sharply in response to exercise, particularly if the exercise is intense. The best way to get your aerobic fitness measured is in a lab or gym, but there are also ways to do it yourself, which we outline at the back of the book.

## Glucose tolerance

In 1922 three scientists called Banting, Best and Collip went into a ward full of comatose and dying children. They injected each child with a substance recently extracted from the pancreas of a calf foetus. Before they had reached the last child the first children were already coming out of their comas. Their parents, who had been told nothing could be done, wept in shocked delight. It was a glorious moment in the long history of medicine, a miracle. The substance they had injected was insulin.

The reason those children were in a coma was because they had Type 1 diabetes. They were dying because their bodies could no longer produce enough insulin. As a result their blood sugar levels had risen out of control.

Prior to the identification, extraction and purification of insulin there was little that could be done for children with Type 1 diabetes. They became intensely hungry and thirsty before slipping into a coma and dying. The only treatment that appeared to make any difference was severe calorie restriction.

The villain was glucose. Glucose is an essential part of our lives, the main fuel that our cells use for energy. But glucose is also toxic. Persistently high levels are associated with all sorts of unpleasant consequences, ranging from increased risk of diabetes, blindness, kidney failure and heart disease to amputation, cancer, dementia and death.

Fortunately, most of us have a pancreas that will respond to a surge in glucose by pumping out insulin. Insulin is a sugar controller; it aids the extraction of glucose from blood and then stores it in places like your liver or muscles in a stable form called glycogen, to be used if and when it is needed.

What is less commonly known is that insulin is also a fat controller. It inhibits lipolysis, the release of stored body fat. At the same time, it forces fat cells to take up and store fat from your blood. High levels of insulin lead to increased fat storage, low levels to fat depletion.

The trouble with a Western diet, drenched in fat and

sugary, carbohydrate-rich foods and drinks, is that it forces your pancreas to pump out ever increasing quantities of insulin. Up to a point this magnificent organ will cope, but ultimately it will simply give up. You are now a diabetic.

Rates of diabetes worldwide have increased tenfold in the last decade and there are now at least 285 million diabetics, most of them Type 2. Unlike type 1, which normally occurs in childhood, Type 2 is largely a result of being overweight and inactive. By 2030 at least 500 million people are expected to be diagnosed as diabetic, with the same number undiagnosed.

## Why blood sugar levels matter to everyone, not just diabetics

Though we don't know it, many of us have persistently high levels of both glucose and insulin which, while they are not in the diabetic range, are nonetheless an indicator of future problems.

Excess glucose in the blood – that is, glucose which has not been taken up by our cells – binds to body proteins (a process called glycation), damaging arteries and nerves. It also makes us look older. In a recent study[8] 600 men and women had their blood glucose levels measured and then, on the basis of their photos, had their age estimated. Diabetics and those with higher blood sugar levels were perceived as being significantly older than they were. This is probably because excess glucose attacks collagen and elastin, proteins that help make skin look supple and youthful.

One of the more important measures of your biological fitness is how swiftly and effortlessly your body is able to get your blood glucose back down to safe levels. See the back of the book for more details.

Although most forms of exercise will improve your aerobic and metabolic fitness, intensity seems to be particularly important for improving both. Intensity also matters when it comes to weight loss.

## The weight-loss fallacy – why long and slow is not the way to go

One of the main reasons we take up exercise is because we have been led to believe that it will help us lose weight. We stand on the scales, gulp, and join the gym. We go a few times a week, and pound away on the treadmill or the exercise bike. The whole thing probably takes a couple of hours, by the time we have travelled there and back, had a shower, had a chat. But we feel virtuous. At the end of our first week we optimistically get back on the scales.

No change.

Ah well, obviously haven't been doing it for long enough, must keep going. So we continue going to the gym and at the end of a month discover that, despite all that time and effort, there has again been little change on the scales.

How is this possible? It is so unfair. We have been repeatedly told that if we do the exercise we will reap the reward, but we don't see any difference. It is at this point that our motivation slumps as we fail to see results and we realise we are going to have to put in hour after hour of slog for minimal gain. And then, like many before us who started out at the gym with good intentions, we give up.

If this happens to you then take some small consolation from the fact that you are not alone. As Dr Stephen Boutcher of the School of Medical Sciences at the University of New South Wales has said, 'Most exercise programmes designed for weight loss have focused on steady state exercise of around 30 minutes at a moderate intensity on most days of the week. Disappointingly, these kinds of exercise programmes have led to little or no loss.'[9]

In the aerobic workout heyday of the 1980s and 90s it was universally accepted that we burn more calories from fat when working at lower intensities. Go steady, but go long, was the advice, and you will enter the 'fat-burning zone'. Jump on any older piece of cardio equipment and you'll see that the lower heart rate zone is still labelled 'fat burning'.

The truth is, however, that, although you will burn

some fat at low intensity, it won't be much and it won't make a significant dent in your paunch.

So why doesn't moderate intensity exercise do what it is supposed to do, what we have been promised it will do? It should be straightforward. Do more exercise, burn more calories, lose more weight.

The problem is that, when it comes to humans, things are rarely straightforward.

Let's look at what happened in a study done at the University of Pittsburgh[10] where they followed nearly 200 overweight women for 2 years while they went through an intensive weight-loss programme. The women were asked to make a big cut in their calorie intake – they had to consume less than 1500 calories a day – and to significantly increase their exercise levels.

To make sure the women kept to the programme they got lots of support. They were given treadmills to take home, they were encouraged to meet frequently and they had regular phone calls urging them to keep going.

Initially, all went well. Six months after starting the programme, more than half the women had lost at least 10% of their body weight and most were still doing regular exercise. Then, as often happens, things began to fall apart. Most of the women lapsed and started to regain the weight they had so painfully lost. Some did manage to keep going to the 2-year mark, but to keep the weight off they were having to do significant amounts of exercise, nearly 70 minutes a day, 5 days a week.

So why is it so difficult to shed fat? Well, part of the problem is that fat is an incredibly energy-dense substance. A pound of fat contains more energy than a pound of dynamite. This means you have to do a lot of exercise to burn even a small amount of fat.

To find out just how much, I returned to Loughborough University where I was put through my paces by sports scientist Dr Keith Tolfrey.

Keith asked me to wear a facemask attached to mobile monitoring equipment. The equipment, he told me, would measure the amount of oxygen I breathed in and the amount of carbon dioxide I breathed out. From that he could calculate the number of calories I burnt while running.

Keith got me to run at a brisk pace around the track, while he cycled alongside shouting encouragement. I wasn't exactly going at Olympic pace, but I was going fast enough to feel relieved when, after 10 minutes, Keith told me I could stop.

Then he and his colleagues gathered around the data gathering machine and announced that I had consumed around 14 calories a minute, which meant that, having run a mile, I had burnt through a grand total of... 140 calories. Not bad, I thought. But put it in perspective. A small bar of chocolate contains about 240 calories, while a large chocolate muffin comes in at an impressive 520 calories. So if you decide to have a muffin and a medium latte (150 calories) after your run, then you are topping yourself up with 670 calories.

And it gets worse, because the figures I just gave you are misleading. When you are judging the benefits of exercise you really should take into account that you would also be burning quite a lot of calories just by sitting down. The fact is that most of the calories we burn come from simply keeping our bodies going. So what you want to know is not the total calorie burn (TBC) but the net calorie burn (NCB), i.e. how many extra calories you burn by running rather than lying on the sofa. Funnily enough, you are rarely given this net figure. Perhaps because it might be discouraging.

To calculate your NCB from running a mile at a reasonable pace (doing 6 miles an hour, say, or walking at about 3mph), use these formulae:

NCB from running a mile at moderate pace = 0.7 x your weight (in lb)

NCB for walking a mile at around 3mph = 0.4 x your weight (in lb)

If you compare these figures with those you will find at popular websites, where they only give you the TCB, you will see they are rather lower.[11]

The one consoling fact about these formulae is that the heavier you are the more calories you will get through. When I did the run with Keith, I weighed 180lb, which meant that my NCB from running a mile was about 126 calories. Since then I have dropped to 160lb (through Intermittent Fasting), so I would now burn through 112 calories while covering the same distance.

My wife, who is 120lb, would get through just 78 calories running a mile, 48 calories walking a mile. Life is unfair.

Let's look at how far would she would have to run or walk to burn through some common snacks or drinks.

|  | CALORIES | RUNNING | WALKING |
|---|---|---|---|
| Banana | 90 | 1.1 miles | 40 mins |
| Glass apple juice | 120 | 1.5 miles | 50 mins |
| Small glass wine/175ml | 126 | 1.6 miles | 1 hour |
| Smoothie/250ml | 140-180 | 2 miles | 1 hour 20 mins |
| Tall latte | 180 | 2.2 miles | 1 hour 30 mins |
| Small chocolate bar | 240 | 3 miles | 1 hour 40 mins |
| Large chocolate muffin | 480 | 6 miles | 3 hrs 20 mins |

You can begin to see the difficulty of trying to lose weight through exercise alone.

There are roughly 3500 calories in a pound of fat, which means that to shed a single pound of fat through exercise I would need to run at least an hour a day for 6 days. Or I could run a marathon. Either way, it is a lot of running.

Running, then, is not a great way of burning calories. What about other forms of exercise, like weight lifting? Dr Jason Gill from Glasgow University has measured the calories you consume while doing this and the results are even less impressive. 'You burn more calories going for a gentle stroll than doing strenuous weight training,' he told me.

'But surely weight training builds muscle and therefore increases your metabolic rate?' I protested.

'Yes, but not much,' replied Jason. 'If you trained hard for 6 months you would probably raise your daily metabolic rate by about 100 calories a day, which is the equivalent of a small glass of fruit juice.'

This was discouraging. And there was more bad news. You might think, 'Perhaps the reason I'm not losing weight despite doing lots of exercise is because I am turning fat into muscle and muscle is, of course, heavier than fat.' Well, that could be true, but then again it probably isn't.

In a recent Australian study,[12] they took 45 overweight young women and randomly allocated them to different exercise regimes. One group was asked to cycle at moderate intensity, 3 times a week, 40 minutes at a time, for 15 weeks. They were properly supervised to make sure they had done their exercise. At the end of the trial, just as they had at the beginning, they underwent a DEXA scan to measure their body fat (for more on DEXA scanning, see page 182). I would not have wanted to be the person who gave them the results, because after 30 hours of cycling they had, on average, put on a pound of fat.

How is this possible? Surely there must have been some mistake? Well, no, there is a painful but very obvious explanation. Studies show that when we begin to exercise most of us don't stick to our normal food intake. We often compensate by eating more. Sometimes a lot more. In fact, even the *thought* of exercise may encourage us to start eating.

In a study done at the University of Illinois, students were asked to evaluate the effectiveness of some lifestyle leaflets. The students were split into 2 groups. One group looked at leaflets encouraging them to do more exercise, the other group at leaflets which urged them to make friends. Afterwards they were asked to eat raisins, to rate their flavour. The students who had been shown the exercise leaflets ate a third more raisins than the other group.

Now this is hardly a real-world experiment, but there is plenty of evidence from the real world that we are prone to compensatory eating.

As Dr Gill told me, 'The initial effects of exercise are often to decrease appetite. The trouble is, we may decide to reward ourselves after a heavy session in the gym with a bar of chocolate or a full-fat cappuccino. There is evidence that we unconsciously eat to fill the energy gap, or compensate for increased activity by doing less when we are not exercising.'

## A brief explanation of Set Point Theory

The studies which suggest that your body will unconsciously try to sabotage your attempts to lose fat are supported by something called Set Point Theory. This theory is an attempt to explain why it is that so many people who try to lose weight through exercise, dieting or some combination of the two, find it hard. The answer seems to be that your body will do all it can to keep your weight steady, at a particular set point.

Imagine you are overweight and decide to lose a few pounds. You go on a diet and increase the amount of exercise you do. Initially the weight drops off. Great. Then it slows. You have cut your calories and increased your activity but not much is happening. What's going on?

Well, as you lose weight your metabolic rate slows down, simply because you are carrying around less weight than you were before. But the amount your metabolic rate slows cannot be explained simply by weight loss. It seems that your body also becomes more efficient at storing and using calories.

The good news is that exercise will slow the rate at which your metabolic rate falls. The bad news is that it isn't as effective as we once hoped.

In a review study, published in 2012, researchers asked plaintively, 'Why do individuals not lose more weight from an exercise intervention?'[13]

The answer seems to be three-pronged: it's because even the experts underestimate how much exercise is needed to shift fat; because the volunteers in these studies compensate by eating more; and finally because exercise has less effect on keeping your metabolic rate revved up than previously believed.

This study was carried out at Penning Biomedical Research Center, where they have created an interesting and hopefully more accurate weight-loss predictor which you can use at: http://www.pbrc.edu/research-and-faculty/calculators/weight-loss-predictor/

Based on this calculator, I can see that, if I start running for an hour a day, 5 days a week (without compensatory eating), then I will lose around 3lb in the first month. Not bad. But unless I increase the length or intensity of my run this rate of loss will soon slow. By the end of 6 months, my exercise regime will lead to about half that weight loss i.e. 1.5lb a month. By the end of 12 months it's helping me lose just 0.1lb a week. Effectively nothing.

## So should I give up now?

Although this may all sound defeatist and gloomy there is good news as well.

For starters, there are benefits to exercise that go beyond weight. From a health point of view it is better to be fat and fit than lean and not fit.

In a study done at the Cooper Institute in Dallas, Texas,[14] researchers followed 22,000 men, aged between 30 and 83, for more than 8 years. Before the study started the men had a full medical check-up, including a treadmill exercise test which tested their aerobic fitness. Over the 8 years of follow-up, 427 of the men died, mainly from heart disease and cancer.

What they discovered in this study is that, when it comes to living longer, fitness is more important than fatness. The men who were overweight but fit were far less likely to die than the men who were normal weight but unfit. In fact, a fit overweight man was no more likely to die than a fit man of normal weight. (A similar study published in 2006 showed that the same is true of women.)

So if you want to live a long and healthy life it seems that being fit is more important than being slim.

Another thing about exercise is that although on its own it is not a great way of losing weight, when you combine it with a diet the combination is likely to be more effective than either done alone.

In a recently published study by Krista Varady and other researchers from the University of Illinois in Chicago,[15] 64 obese volunteers were randomly allocated to 1 of 4 groups: either ADF (alternate day fasting – i.e. eating a quarter of their normal calorie intake every other day) plus endurance exercise; ADF alone; endurance exercise alone; or a control group.

After 12 weeks, those doing ADF plus exercise had lost 6kg (just over 13lb), compared to 3kg (6.5lb) for ADF alone and 1kg (just over 2lb) for exercise alone. Those doing the combined approach also saw the biggest improvements in cholesterol and fat loss. The researchers concluded that exercise plus dieting 'produces superior changes in body weight, body composition, and lipid indicators of heart disease risk, when compared to individual treatments'.

## In summary

Exercise is clearly good for us – it's good for our mood, our general health and our brains – but it is not a guaranteed way of losing weight. This is because:

- Traditional low intensity exercise is not a time-efficient way of burning fat

- If you are going to lose weight and keep it off, exercise is not enough on its own – you also have to curb calories

- After a bout of exercise, there is a tendency to indulge in a bout of compensatory eating. Try not to undo the good you have done through exercising by rewarding yourself with a high-calorie snack

- We are also more likely to reduce the amount of activity we do after exercising. Look out for compensatory slacking...

Fret not! It is possible to get fitter and lose fat. Read on.

# WHAT IS FAST EXERCISE?

There is a persistent widespread belief in the fitness industry that the more time you spend exercising, the better. Only those who dedicate themselves to punishingly lengthy workouts can expect their body fat to plummet, their muscles to become exquisitely defined, to finally enter the kingdom of heavenly bodies. Tracey Anderson, trainer to Gwyneth Paltrow and Jennifer Lopez, famously said that she expects devotees of her method to spend 90 minutes a day on her regime. Madonna reportedly spends 2 hours a day with her trainer.

If that is how you wish to spend your time, good luck. If not, then you will be pleased to hear that the question occupying the minds of many of those at the forefront of exercise research is not so much 'How can we get people to do more?' but 'How can we get more for less'. HIT has caused a stir because studies done over the last decade have repeatedly shown that a few minutes of intense exercise a day can make a significant difference.

Yet the principles behind HIT are not new. Not even remotely new.

# How the hunter-gatherers did it

Each of us has a deep history. We are the product of thousands of generations of our species, a species that for most of its existence has lived precariously. Life for a caveman or woman was generally nasty, brutish and short. To keep in shape they didn't 'exercise'; they simply did a wide range of different activities that helped ensure that they survived and passed on their genes, eventually, to us. Our bodies and our genes were forged by the demands of the environment in which they lived. Perhaps by looking to the past we can learn how to stay in shape, and ensure that we have a future.

The problem, of course, is that our Pleistocene ancestors are long gone and it is impossible to say with great accuracy and simply by looking at their remains how they would have lived. The closest examples we have today of people who live much as our ancestors may have done are hunter-gatherers, people like the Hadza of northern Tanzania.

The Hadza live very near the Olduvai Gorge, part of the Great Rift Valley. Due to the large number of very ancient human fossils that have been found in the area it is sometimes known as the 'Cradle of Mankind'. In the surrounding land there is evidence of hominid occupation going back nearly 2 million years, including indications of *Homo erectus*, *Homo habilis* and early *Homo sapiens*.

Hunter gatherers have been living in the area for at least 50,000 years and for much of that time the ancestors of the Hadza have been left untouched by 'civilisation'. Until recently, the Hadza still hunted on foot using bows, axes and digging sticks. They did not have cars or guns. They certainly did not have access to fast-food joints or gyms.

For some reason I had this idea that hunter-gatherers spend a lot of time travelling at a gentle jog, tracking game for days on end. In fact, when anthropologists started following the Hadza, they found that they don't do a lot unless they have to. In a study in which they asked the Hadza to wear GPS trackers and other sophisticated sensors, they found that, contrary to what you might expect, the number of calories they burn per pound of body weight is about the same as yours or mine.[16]

The reason they don't run about much is that they live on a relatively low-calorie diet. They need to conserve their energy. Instead of jogging, the men typically walk about 7 miles (11km) a day while hunting food. Women, who are less involved in hunting, cover more like 4 miles (6km) a day. Both sexes do energy-sapping tasks like chopping wood and digging up tubers to eat, but they also do a lot of loafing around. Not surprisingly, they tend to be lean: a Hadza man in his mid-thirties typically has a body-fat percentage of 13%, a woman one of around 21%. This compares to the average in North America of 21% for men and 34% for women.

What is clear from studying hunter-gatherers is that

they do a proper mix of different activities. They alternate low intensity but fairly constant movement with short bursts of high intensity activity (i.e. hunting, climbing trees, chopping wood). They also alternate periods of strenuous activity with days where they do relatively little.

As we'll show, there is compelling evidence that this hunter-gatherer approach is also good for our more cosseted bodies. We need to be active, but not too active. We benefit from short bursts of intense activity and we need rest days to recover or we undo all the good work. As the authors of 'Achieving Hunter-gatherer fitness in the 21st Century', a paper in the *American Journal of Medicine*,[17] point out,

'Hunter-gatherers would have likely alternated difficult days with less demanding days when possible. The same pattern of alternating a strenuous workout one day with an easy one the next day produces higher levels of fitness with lower rates of injury... The natural cross-training that was a mandatory aspect of life as a hunter-gatherer improves performance across many athletic disciplines.'

In fact, the authors are so convinced that a hunter-gatherer lifestyle is beneficial that they put together what they call 'The characteristics of a Hunter-gatherer Fitness Programme'. According to this, if you want to exercise like a hunter-gatherer, you should:

1. Do a lot of light background activity such as walking.
2. Have hard days followed by easy days. You need rest, relaxation and sleep.
3. Include interval training: short intermittent bursts of moderate to high intensity exercise interspersed with rest and recovery, 2-3 times a week.
4. Make sure you do regular sessions of strength- and flexibility-building. Hunter-gatherers have to chop wood, climb trees or carry a child around.
5. Ideally do all exercise outdoors, where you get exposed to sunlight, which gives your skin a chance to generate vitamin D. Although it is called a vitamin, 'vitamin' D is actually a hormone, with a far wider range of activity than people had previously imagined. Many of us, particularly those who live in the northern hemisphere, are chronically short of vitamin D.
6. Try to do as much exercise as possible in a social setting. We are intensely social creatures and doing exercise together is a good way of ensuring that we do it at all.

Fast Exercise is based on the hunter-gatherer approach. In Chapter 3, Peta offers a range of workouts that use different forms of HIT, many of which can be done outdoors; and in Chapter 5, I describe ways in which you can build more activity into your life. But before we come to that, let's look at the story behind the discovery of HIT.

## A short history of HIT

One of the first people to use high intensity interval training and to study it scientifically was an early 20th-century German coach called Woldemar Gerschler. He was, by all accounts, an extremely demanding man, but a man who was passionately interested in the science of exercise.

The athletes that trained with him were typically asked to sprint 100, 200, sometimes 400 metres at a pace that would get their hearts up to 180 beats per minute. They would then wait till their heart rate dropped to 120, before doing it again. Gerschler had realised that it was the combination of intensity and recovery that was critical.

Gerschler showed that in less than 3 weeks he could increase an athlete's heart volume by 20% and make significant improvements in their race times. His students began to put together some truly remarkable performances.

In 1939 Rudolf Harbig, a runner coached by Gerschler,

broke the world 800-metre record by a massive 1.6 seconds. The following month he broke the world 400-metre record as well. His 800-metre record lasted 16 years, until in 1955 Roger Moens, an athlete who was also coached by Gerschler, ran it in 1:45.7.

Meanwhile, in 1950s Britain, a young medical student, Roger Bannister, was determined to become the first person in the world to run a sub-4-minute mile. The trouble was, as a busy student he didn't have lots of spare time for training. So he would go down to the track and do interval sprints. These consisted of running flat out for about 1 minute, during which time he would cover a quarter of a mile (440 yards, about 400 metres). Then he would jog for 2-3 minutes before doing another one-minute sprint. He would repeat this cycle 10 times, then head back to work. Since he rarely bothered with much in the way of warm-ups or cool-downs, the whole thing normally took less than 35 minutes.

In May 1954, Roger Bannister took part in a race at the Iffley Road track in Oxford, which he duly won. The announcer, Norris McWhirter (who went on to co-edit the *Guinness Book of Records*), clearly enjoyed his share of what would turn out to be a great sporting moment. Slowly, ponderously, he spelt out the results: 'Ladies and gentlemen, here is the result of event 9, the one mile: 1st, No. 41, R.G. Bannister, Amateur Athletic Association and formerly of Exeter and Merton Colleges, Oxford, with a time which is a new meeting and track record, and which – subject to ratification – will be a new English Native, British National, All-Comers, European, British Empire and World Record. The time was 3...'

There was a huge roar which drowned out the rest of the message as the crowd realised that the '3...' must mean they had just watched the first person to run the mile in less than 4 minutes.

What I find particularly interesting about this story is that Roger Bannister's regime – 10 sets of 1-minute sprints, split by a couple of minutes of recovery – is now widely used by HIT enthusiasts, and not, as we'll see, just by serious runners but by the overweight, the unfit and those with previous histories of cardiac problems. It is also the way that Peta likes to train.

Other incredibly successful middle-distance athletes have used different HIT regimes. Sebastian Coe, who once held world records in the 800 metres, the mile and the 1500 metres at the same time, did fast sprints with short recoveries, but in his case it was more likely to be 20-second sprints with 30 seconds' recovery. That is my preferred regime, too – though I do it on a bicycle and only manage to do it about 3 times before collapsing.

## HIT and elite athletes

When Coe was breaking world records in the 1970s, HIT was still relatively little used and seen mainly as a way of increasing speed, not endurance. These days there is unlikely to be any athlete who has reached the top in any sport without having made this sort of exercise at least part of their workload.

It's pretty obvious that athletes who engage in sports that require stop-start bursts of speed – tennis, football, squash, hockey and martial arts – will benefit from HIT. In many ways the HIT approach simulates what they will experience in competition – including the build-up of waste products in tired limbs and the need to override those almost crippling effects to be able to sprint again. And again. And again.

Cyclists, sprinters and swimmers who compete in shorter distance races have to learn to push themselves to the limit in one training session, but ensure that their bodies have recovered for the next. For all of these, HIT-type training several times a week is a tried and tested solution.

What is more surprising is how important HIT is for endurance athletes. For elite long-distance cyclists, marathon runners, triathletes, race-walkers and open-water swimmers, variations of HIT increasingly form a big part of their training programme. HIT – by putting the body under stress and increasing mitochondrial activity (which we'll come to in depth later) – adds to explosive power.

In short, HIT allows athletes to run, swim and cycle faster for longer. It prepares them for the discomfort that comes from extremes of effort and primes their bodies to deal with the worst that high-level competition can throw at them. And to finish on top.

## What about the rest of us?

The trouble with trying to extrapolate from studies with trained athletes is that these people are, almost by definition, unlike the rest of us. What can HIT do for us lesser mortals? Over the last 2 decades lots of researchers around the world have studied the effects of HIT in different populations, but the man who has done more than most is Martin Gibala, Professor of Exercise Science at McMaster University in Canada.

Back in 2005, he and his colleagues published a study which had a huge impact on the exercise world.[18]

They asked 8 reasonably active young volunteers to do six sessions of what they called SIT – sprint interval training. Training consisted of between 4 and 7 sessions, carried out over 2 weeks, with 1-2 days rest in between each session.

SIT is real misnomer. It sounds easy. It is not. You get on a special bike and, after a brief warm-up, you have to cycle flat out for 30 seconds against resistance. You then have a breather that lasts about 4 minutes, which you spend gently pedalling, then you do another 30-second sprint. Gradually you build it up. When the brave volunteers did it back in the mid-1990s, they were doing this up to 7 times in each session.

It is difficult to imagine how tough this really is. The first 30-second burst is OK. You think to yourself, 'That was manageable.' The next 30-second burst is hard. You really welcome the 4-minute break. The third time, you cannot believe how slowly the seconds go past. The pedals slow; you have to focus to try and keep up speed. By the time you get to number 7 (if you ever get to number 7) you are truly knackered and need to lie down on the sofa for a while.

SIT is tiring, but the time commitment is very low. In total the SIT volunteers did only 15 minutes of hard exercise across the 2 weeks and those 15 minutes made some impressive differences.

The volunteers' 'cycle endurance capacity', their ability to push themselves hard on a bike, doubled. Whereas previously they had managed to cycle hard for 26 minutes, now they could do it for 51 minutes. Something remarkable had gone on inside their bodies.

But what?

Martin Gibala did another study.[19]

This time he decided (or his volunteers told him) that doing 7 lots of 30 seconds per session was too much for a normal human to endure. So he generously cut it down to a maximum of 6.

He enlisted 16 young men (these studies are often but not exclusively done with men, probably because men are more likely to be found hanging around science labs) and randomly divided them into 2 groups.

Eight were asked to do 6 sessions of cycling at reasonable intensity for 1½ to 2 hours at a time.

The other group also did 6 sessions, but with short bursts of flat-out cycling. In each session they did 2-3 minutes of intense exercise, which along with the recovery periods meant each session lasted about 20 minutes.

At the end of training the steady-cycling volunteers had spent more than 10 hours on their bikes, while the SIT lot had done just over 2 hours.

When researchers did the the follow-up tests (including muscle biopsies, which I can tell you from personal experience is not pleasant), they found that both groups had improved on a whole range of measures by much the same amount. The difference was that it had taken the SIT group a fifth of the time.

## *Making it easier: the Bannister method*

By now, Martin and his colleagues realised that doing 30-second bursts of flat-out cycling would be a challenge for people who were not already pretty fit. SIT, as Martin explained, 'is extremely demanding and it may not be safe, tolerable or appealing for some individuals'.

So they broke it down further, into a protocol that they believed could be safely done by people who are unfit, overweight or have a previous history of heart disease, stroke or diabetes.[20]

The new protocol consisted of doing 10 bursts of 1-minute sprints, separated by 1 minute of recovery. This sort of protocol is somewhat similar to the one I described earlier, used by Roger Bannister when he was training to break the 4-minute mile.

The main difference is that during those 1-minute sprints you are not going flat out. Instead you should be aiming to cycle hard enough to raise your pulse to about 80-90% of your maximal heart rate (to find out how to calculate this, see the 'Ways to Measure the Impact of Exercise' section at the back). From my experience it is tough but bearable. It is also delightfully brief.

## So how does HIT work, and what difference does it make?

There have been dozens of studies of different forms of HIT. Most have been quite short (a couple of weeks); some have lasted a few months. And so far only a few hundred people have been intensively studied (though the results of some big studies are expected soon).

Nonetheless, what the studies done so far consistently show is that:

- HIT will get you aerobically fitter faster than standard exercise

- HIT will improve insulin sensitivity faster than standard exercise

- If you want to build muscle tone and lose some fat HIT is the most time-efficient way to achieve this

Let's look at the science behind HIT, and how it actually works.

## Mitochondria or power cells

One of the reasons why doing HIT produces big changes in a short time is because of the effect that high intensity exercise has on your mitochondria.

Mitochondria are the body's main power plants. Their job is to convert raw materials like oxygen and glucose into little packages of energy called ATP (adenosine triphosphate). The ATP is then used to power your body.

But mitochondria are much more than that. As Nick Lane puts it in his 2005 book, *Power, Sex, Suicide*, they are the 'clandestine rulers of the world'. Despite the fact that they are so small (a billion could fit in a grain of sand), they are the great turbo-chargers of life, responsible for the extraordinary range of creatures that live on earth today, including us.

There are mitochondria in every cell of your body, ranging from a few to many thousands. They are unlike anything else in your body because they have their own DNA, which is closer to that of bacteria than to that of human beings. They are interlopers, aliens, yet they are essential to our existence. Their long and fascinating history is, I think, worth a brief digression.

If we could travel back a few billion years, we would discover a profoundly different Earth. The days would be shorter, the atmosphere almost devoid of oxygen and the continents would be completely unrecognisable. There would be no trees, no plants, no animals. In fact, the only forms of life you would encounter would be tiny single-celled microbes. These microbes got their energy through fermentation, breaking down complex compounds, and thrived in the anaerobic (oxygen-free) atmosphere of ancient Earth.

Then, around 2 billion years ago, a new creature appeared. It was a microbe with a difference, one that would change everything. This new microbe had acquired the ability to use sunlight as a source of power. It was a microbe that could photosynthesise.

Unfortunately for the other microscopic creatures that was living on our planet, generating energy through photosynthesis led to the release of an extremely toxic gas as a by-product. Over tens of millions of years the levels of this poisonous gas increased from virtually nothing to almost 21% of the entire atmosphere. It was the worst outbreak of pollution that this world has ever known and resulted in the death of countless life forms.

The by-product of photosynthesis was, of course, oxygen – and the effects of its increased levels in the atmosphere were so dramatic that the period has been labelled the Oxygen Catastrophe or Oxygen Crisis.

What the new super-microbes that 'invented' photo-synthesis had done was use energy from sunlight to split water ($H_2O$) into oxygen and hydrogen. They mixed hydrogen with carbon to make simple sugars – i.e. food – the oxygen was just released into the atmosphere.

While we think of oxygen as life-giving, it's actually extremely toxic. It reacts hungrily with proteins and enzymes, stopping them from working.; it causes metal to rust. If levels rose much above where they are at present, trees would burst spontaneously into flames.

The reason why oxygen levels didn't simply go on rising is that eventually a new breed of microbes evolved an even smarter chemical trick – they learnt how to convert oxygen, the great poison, into energy.

The microbes that did this were an early ancestor of the tiny mitochondria that now live happily inside our cells. We have acquired, though them, the ability to use oxygen as a fuel. We can also, thanks to even earlier microscopic ancestors, produce energy anaerobically, i.e. without oxygen, though this is a far less efficient process. So when people talk about doing aerobic exercise they are really talking about doing a form of exercise that depends primarily on getting mitochondria to produce power.

I've gone on at length about mitochondria because they are important for understanding how HIT works. Since mitochondria produce power, then, broadly speaking, you want more of them. One way to produce more is to do exercise. In fact, a good measure of how effective an exercise regime is going to be is whether it results in greater mitochondrial density.

And that's where HIT seems to score particularly well. Doing HIT leads to the production of greater numbers of more active mitochondria than doing standard exercise will. This is true not just in skeletal muscle (i.e. the muscles that make you move) but also heart muscle (the muscle that keeps you alive).

HIT makes heart muscle bigger and more efficient. After doing HIT your heart muscle needs less oxygen to do the same amount of work. In short, doing HIT leads to a bigger, stronger heart.

This is important because one of the main fears about doing HIT is that it could trigger a heart attack or stroke. In fact, there is convincing evidence that doing HIT will *reduce* the risk of this happening and will also help you recover faster after a heart attack. It's a promising but still controversial area of research which I will return to later.

## Fast Exercise and fat

The other good thing about mitochondria is that they burn fat. So if HIT makes more mitochondria it should lead to more fat burning. But what's the evidence? Well, let's return once more to the Australian study – in which 45 women were randomly allocated to either 3 x 40 minutes of moderate intensity cycling a week (see page 46) or three 20-minute sessions of higher intensity intermittent cycling.[21]

The women who had been allocated to the high intensity group were asked to alternate 8 seconds of sprint cycling with 12 seconds of gentle cycling. They started doing this for 5 minutes, building up to 20 minutes per session.

At the end of 15 weeks, both groups had got fitter, as measured by improvements in their aerobic fitness, or VO2 max, but only the high intensity group had lost any weight. They lost an average of 2.5kg (5.5lb) – but within this average there was huge variability. Some of the women lost up to 8kg (17.6lb), a few lost very little. The ones who lost very little were the ones who were lean to begin with. The fatter the women were at the start of the study, the more fat they had lost by the end.

However, the women who did normal moderate intensity cycling, despite spending twice as long on their bikes, managed to put on weight and became slightly fatter.

The particularly good news from this study was that the women doing the HIT lost fat not only from their thighs, which you might expect, but also from their stomachs. The reduction in abdominal fat was accompanied by a decrease in fasting insulin, down by 31%.

If you were wondering if the same is true of men, the research team did a similar study using young overweight males. They recruited 46 inactive, overweight young men (aged around 25) and got them to do three 20-minute sessions a week on an exercise bike. Like the women, after a brief warm-up, they had to sprint for 8 seconds, then cycle gently for 12 seconds. The idea was to try and keep their heart rate racing along at around 80-90% of maximum while sprinting. In men this age that would mean pushing the heart rate up to around 160 beats per minute.[22]

After 6 weeks there was not much change in body fat, which must have been discouraging. Then, however, the changes really began to kick in. By the end of 12 weeks the young men's aerobic power had increased by 15% and on average they had lost 2kg (4.4lb) of fat. Encouragingly they had lost a lot of that fat from the gut (visceral fat was down by 17%) and they had put on muscle.

Compared to the Australian women who had done a

similar regime they put on far more muscle, particularly in the thighs. They had also managed to do it in less time, as this trial ran for 12 weeks rather than 15.

In another study from the University of Ontario,[23] 10 men and 10 women were randomly allocated to do HIT or to do lengthy runs 3 times a week for 6 weeks. Unlike the Australian volunteers, who did 8 seconds of intense cycling followed by 12 seconds' dawdling, this lot were asked to perform 4-6 bursts of 30-second sprints with a recovery period of 4 minutes between each burst.

The control group was asked to run steadily on a treadmill for 60 minutes at a steady pace that raised their heart rate to around 65% of maximum.

At the end of the trial, the steady runners had lost some body fat, but the HIT exercisers had shed more than twice as much, an impressive 12.4% of their fat mass. And they had done it in a fraction of the time.


## How does turning up the HIT burn fat?

★ When you push the intensity of a workout, you build more metabolically active muscle, and because muscle is efficient at burning fat your total calorie expenditure soars. This happens mainly because HIT makes the muscle cells produce new and more active mitochondria, power plants that transfer fat into energy and heat. The mitochondria not only burn fat when you are exercising but go on doing so for some time afterwards as your muscles recover.

★ The metabolic stress caused by HIT also leads to a huge increase in the production of catecholamines – hormones like adrenaline and noradrenaline – that lead to much greater fat burning. As Dr John Babraj and Dr Ross Lorimer point out in their book, *The High Intensity Workout*: 'Adrenaline and noradrenaline are elevated by as much as 1450% following a high intensity training session. The size of the response is much bigger than is seen with steady exercise such as jogging or cycling.'

★ So why does HIT lead to fat loss in your gut? Well one reason is that there are more catecholamine receptors in abdominal fat than in subcutaneous fat, so when you get a surge of catecholamines following a vigorous burst of HIT, they target abdominal fat, increasing the release of fat from visceral fat stores.

★ Catecholamines also activate brown fat (see box below), which burns rather than stores energy.

★ High intensity training also seems to suppress appetite in ways that low intensity exercise does not.

# A note on brown fat

More than 30 years ago I watched a science documentary about something called 'brown fat'. Unlike normal fat, brown fat contains a lot more mitochondria, which is what makes it brown. Brown fat is most commonly found in newborn babies and in hibernating mammals. It is there, primarily, to generate heat. Unlike the more familiar yellowish-white body fat that stores excess calories, brown fat does the opposite. It burns calories. When 'switched on', brown fat produces around 300 times more heat than any other organ in the body.

Back in the 1980s it was thought that activating brown fat would be one way to solve the obesity problem. But things didn't work out so well. Though it had been known for some time that babies have deposits of brown fat around their shoulder blades to help them maintain their body temperature (babies are not very good at shivering), scientists couldn't find brown fat in adults. So they decided brown fat must disappear in infancy once it is no longer really needed. Interest in brown fat dwindled. Recently, thanks to better technology, it has returned.

In the last decade, researchers carrying out PET-CT scans have found traces of brown fat in adults, particularly on the upper back, the side of the neck, in the dip between the collarbone and the shoulder, and along the spine. Not a lot, but enough to encourage further investigation.

It turns out women have proportionately more brown fat than men and it is more readily detectable in lean people than in the obese, although researchers are still not sure why. What's now accepted is that brown fat persists into adulthood and that there are a couple of ways of activating it. What we don't yet know is how big or significant this effect is likely to be.

High intensity exercise certainly leads to a flood of hormones like noradrenaline, known to activate brown fat. Exposure to cold will also encourage your brown fat to burn through a few more calories. Using thermal-imaging techniques, researchers at the University of Nottingham's Queen's Medical Centre have shown that plunging your hands into a bucket of cold water can trigger brown fat into calorie-burning action. Likewise, exercise in the cold can boost the fat-burning effect, one reason to turn the thermostat down and go out for a stroll on a cold winter's night.

## HIT and appetite

Any form of exercise will lead to some fat burning; but, as we've seen already, unless you also curb your calories it will not lead to weight loss. So what effect does HIT have on appetite?

In a trial conducted in 2011,[24] 15 obese adolescent French boys were asked to spend a few days in a metabolic chamber, a room equipped with bed, TV, toilet, exercise bike and not much else. The scientists were able to keep a really close eye on exactly what the boys were up to and what was happening to their metabolisms.

At 8am the boys went into the chamber and ate a carefully measured breakfast. A couple of hours later they were asked to do a session of either high or low intensity cycling (they had to alternate: one day 'high' followed by one day 'low', or vice versa). Whether they were doing high or low intensity cycling, the boys had to keep going until they had burnt off exactly 330 calories.

Thirty minutes after exercising they were offered a buffet lunch, which they tucked into. Buffets are a popular research tool because people just help themselves and are not influenced by the amount of food they are offered.

After lunch the boys were encouraged to be idle for the rest of the day before eating whatever they fancied from a buffet dinner. Then they went to bed.

The boys filled in diaries which showed they didn't notice any difference in their appetite after doing the different levels of exercise nor did they consciously change how much they ate.

Nonetheless, on the days they did high intensity cycling they ate significantly less at the two buffet meals than when they did low intensity exercise.

At lunch, for example, the boys ate 10% less after high intensity exercise than after a less intense session. Even more striking was the buffet dinner, where they ate 20% less than they had on less active days.

The finding from this study is consistent with others which have found that the effects of high intensity exercise on appetite peak around 7 hours after a single bout.

So HIT seems to curb appetite, at least for a while. Unfortunately, the effect of doing HIT does wear off. The following morning (20 hours after exercising) the boys ate just as much breakfast whether they had exercised the previous day or not.

The researchers of this particular study are not entirely sure why high intensity exercise suppresses appetite. They think it might be because of the effect it has on hormones that regulate appetite, such as PYY (see box below), glucagon-like peptide 1 or leptin. They also acknowledge that 'questions still remain as to whether the anorexic effect of HIE [anorexic, as in loss of appetite] can be maintained during prolonged training'.

So, does HIT really lead to long-term appetite suppression? The short answer is that we simply don't know; there have not been sufficient long-term trials yet. But the results from the two Australian studies I mentioned earlier, which ran for 3 months and showed significant fat loss from HIT, suggest it might.

Interestingly, another group of Australian researchers

showed that the more intense the exercise, the longer it suppresses appetite. They took overweight young men in their twenties and early thirties and got them to ride on a stationary bike for 30 minutes, with 1 minute of high intensity cycling followed by 4 minutes of gentle pedalling.

This time, however, they threw in a fourth day when the men had to put themselves through a much tougher version of HIT, cycling for 15 seconds of maximal effort followed by just 1 minute of rest, done for half an hour. They called this very high intensity or VHI.

After each session the men were given a liquid meal containing 300 calories. Then, an hour later, they were offered porridge and told to eat as much as they wanted until they were 'comfortably full'.

Results, published in the *International Journal of Obesity*,[25] showed that the young men ate fewer calories after the high intensity (621 calories) and very high intensity (594 calories) workouts than they did after a bout of moderate exercise (710 calories).

Even more encouragingly, the men reported eating fewer calories on the day *following* the highest intensity workout (2,000 calories) than they did after the moderate session (2,300 calories) or after resting (2,600 calories). As I mentioned above, this suggests that if you do extremely high intensity exercise the effects of appetite suppression last far longer, well into the following day.

They also found some significant differences in the bloods of their volunteers. There were, for example, lower levels of ghrelin, a hunger-promoting hormone, after doing intense exercise than after the gentler versions and there were also higher levels of lactate, which reduces appetite.

Another positive finding was that, although doing HIT was an effort, the men said they had enjoyed the more gruelling version of the exercises.

## HIT and hunger hormones

One of the hottest areas of clinical research, when it comes to weight loss, is the study of hormones produced by your body that control appetite – sometimes referred to as hunger hormones. Ghrelin, for example – a hormone produced by cells in the stomach – seems to increase appetite, while the hormones leptin and peptide YY (also known as PYY) reduce it.

Lots of studies have shown that ghrelin (I remember it as the GREEDY hormone) levels go up before a meal and fall after you have eaten. When you lose weight, average ghrelin levels also tend to rise, encouraging you to eat more and put the weight back on, which is annoying. A bout of insomnia will also make ghrelin levels rise, one reason why chronic sleep shortage can lead to weight gain.

We know that intense exercise will lower your ghrelin levels. What we don't know is how long the effect lasts and whether, in time, your body adjusts.

Leptin has also been intensely studied. Unlike ghrelin, it reduces your appetite. Think of it as the LEAN hormone. Leptin is made in fat tissue and controls your appetite by acting on the hypothalamus, a portion of the brain, suppressing hunger signals. There was, at one time, a widespread hope that a simple injection of leptin would suppress appetite in obese patients and, hey presto, the fat would just melt away. Unfortunately, it has not turned out to be anything like that easy.

Researchers soon discovered that most obese humans are not deficient in leptin. Far from it. They often have extremely high circulating levels of leptin. It seems that once you become obese, your cells become insensitive to leptin, and so your body responds by producing increasing amounts of it. In this respect it is rather like the levels of insulin, which also tend to rise as people become obese and their bodies become increasingly insensitive to its effects.

In the Australian study on young, overweight women outlined in the previous chapter (see page 46), the researchers found that insulin and leptin levels both fell significantly as the women doing HIT lost weight and got fitter. There were no changes in the women doing steady, low intensity exercise.

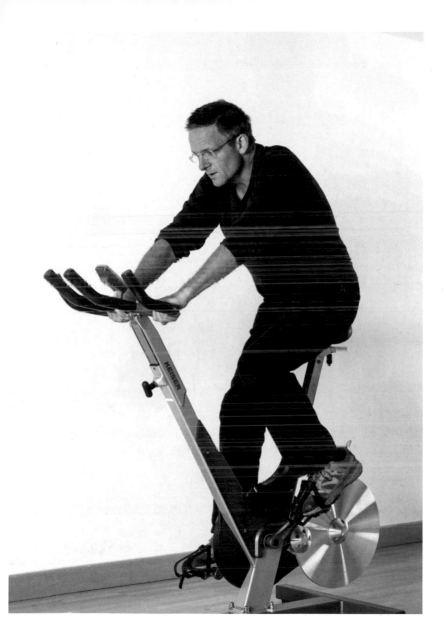

Indoor cycling is a good way of getting HIT: a modern indoor bike lets you add resistance, changing the intensity of the ride.

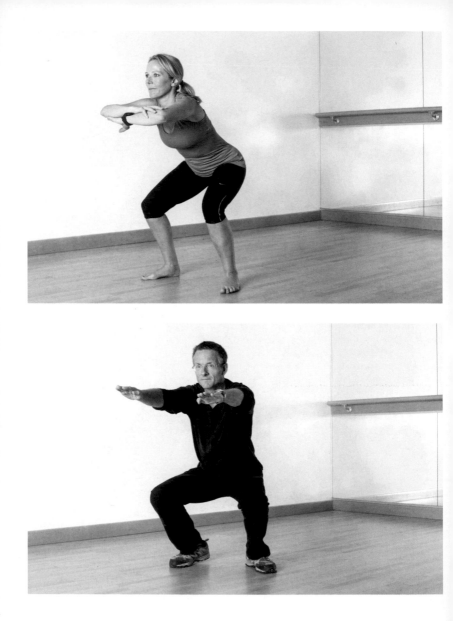

When squatting, bend from the hips, keeping the weight in your heels. Make sure your back is straight. Bend until the legs are at a 90-degree angle – imagine you are preparing to sit in a chair.

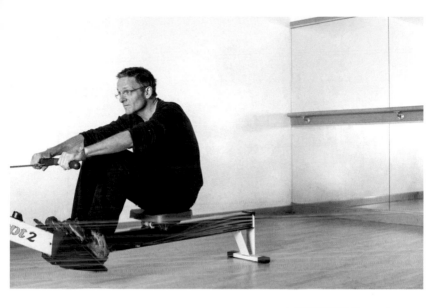

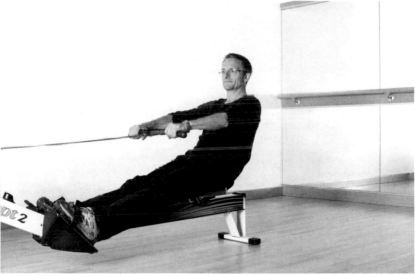

With rowing, good technique is crucial. Start each stroke by pushing with the legs, not pulling with the arms, and keep your wrists in line with the handle so that the pulley wire is parallel to the floor.

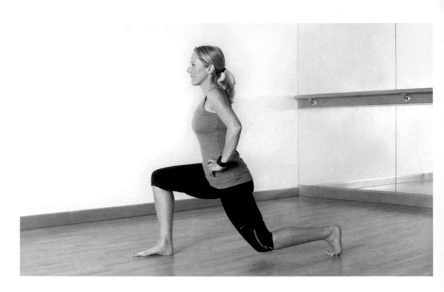

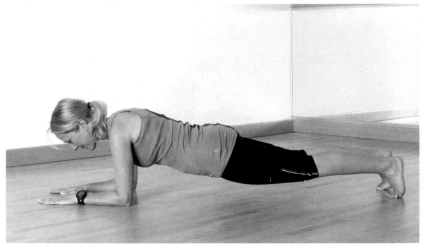

Above, lunges: step forward with one leg, bending both knees to 90 degrees and keeping your upper body straight.

Below, the plank: lift your body off the ground, supporting your weight on your elbows and the balls of your feet. Make sure your mid-section doesn't rise or drop. Hold the position for as long as possible. Remember, it should never cause pain in the lower back.

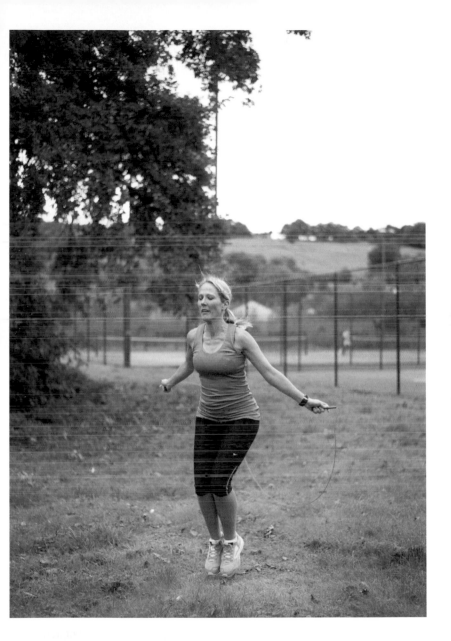

For skipping, knees and ankles should be flexed but your torso kept straight when jumping. Arms should be at your side with the rope turning from the wrists and forearms.

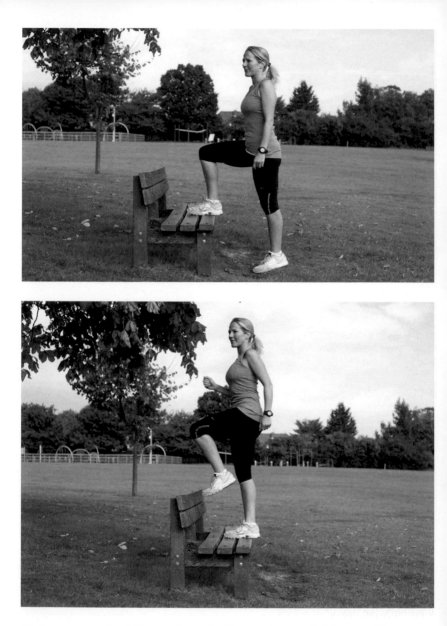

Chair step-ups should be performed with care but at a brisk pace. Place one foot on the 'step', making sure your full foot is in contact with the surface. Push your body weight up, driving your weight through the heel and breathing out as you do this.

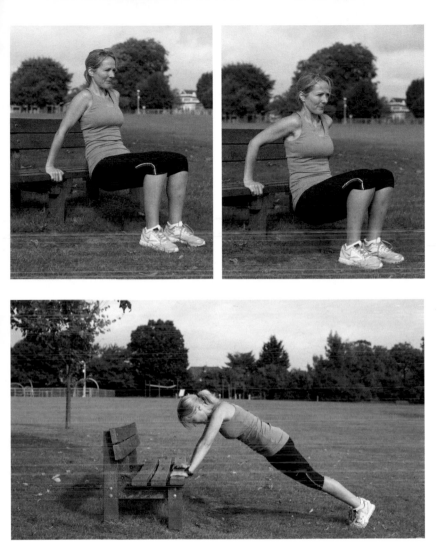

Above, tricep dips: place your palms on the seat behind you, bending your knees at right angles, hips straight. Bend your elbows to 90 degrees to lower your body (so that your bottom descends halfway to the floor).

Below, bench push-ups: be sure to keep your body in a straight line, so that your weight is supported on balls of the feet and by the elbows. Don't allow your back to arch or your hips to drop.

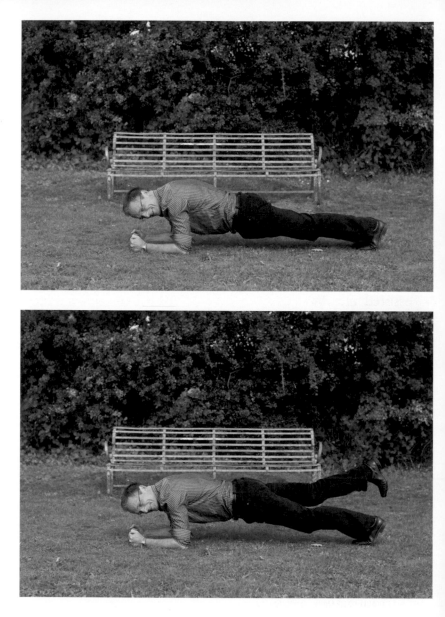

For a plank with leg raise, lift your body off the ground, supporting yourself on your elbows and keeping your back straight. Squeezing the torso tight, slowly lift one foot approximately 6-8 inches off the ground and hold the position for a few seconds.

# My HIT journey

When I first heard about HIT I was curious but sceptical. I liked the idea of getting fit in a short period of time and I particularly liked the idea of improving my insulin sensitivity as my father had died of diabetes-related illnesses and I could see the same thing happening to me.

The form of HIT I decided to start with was 3 bouts of 20 seconds, 3 times a week for 4 weeks. My mentor, Professor Jamie Timmons of Loughborough University, assured me that this sort of regime typically results in improvements in insulin sensitivity of around 25% and increased VO2 max (see page 36) of around 10%. He also warned me that these were average figures, which meant that I might do better than this, or considerably worse.

Before Jamie put me on his short, sharp regime, he measured my glucose tolerance and my VO2 max. I went into the lab, having fasted overnight, and on an empty stomach drank a glass of something with the equivalent of 15 teaspoons of sugar in it. It was disgusting. Then I had to lie down while they took blood samples every 10 minutes for the next 2 hours.

Jamie came to me with the results. I could tell from his face that the news was not particularly good.

'Your results are not perfect,' Jamie said. 'Your blood glucose went up after drinking all that sugar and then it slowly drifted down, just below the level we would call impaired glucose tolerance. So you're just within the healthy range. But only just.'

With that unsettling discovery rattling around inside my head, I got on an exercise bike so they could measure my VO2 max. For the next 20 minutes I pushed myself to my absolute limit, hoping that these results would be a little more encouraging. My VO2 max score, 37mL/(kg·min) – millilitres of oxygen per kilogram of bodyweight per minute – was not outstanding but it was at least acceptable. I would have preferred 'world class' but had to settle for 'good for your age'.

With those results under my belt, I went away to do HIT on a special exercise bike that Jamie lent me. For the next 4 weeks I sprinted my little heart out on that exercise bike for exactly 1 minute a day, 3 days a week. I enjoyed the fact that it was so brief and the challenge of really pushing myself, but I discovered that even 20 seconds at full pelt against resistance can make your thighs burn.

Just to see if it could be done, I sometimes tried doing the sprints in a suit and tie. The answer is yes: because the actual exercise was so brief, I never got uncomfortably hot, let alone sweaty.

After 4 weeks I went back to the lab to be retested. I drank the nauseatingly sweet drink and pushed myself as hard as possible on the bike.

Then it was time for my results. There was good news, and bad news. The good news was that my insulin sensitivity had improved by a remarkable 25%, exactly in line with Jamie's predictions. I was elated, and wondered why this had happened.

Jamie is not exactly sure, but he thinks that one way HIT works is that it disrupts glycogen stores – glucose that's stored in muscles. 'The key thing about this form of exercise is that because it is vigorous it really breaks down the glycogen stores in the muscle and that's a signal from the muscle to the bloodstream saying I need to take up more glucose. Unlike walking or jogging where you may only be activating 20-30% of your muscle tissue, here you're activating 70-80%, so you're really creating a much bigger sink to soak up the glucose that follows a meal.'

That was the good news. My increased insulin sensitivity suggested that I had, for the time being, reduced the risk that I would become a fully-fledged diabetic.

## Me and my glucose

Unless you keep doing it the benefits of any exercise regime will wear off. To find out how quickly, in early 2012 I stopped doing HIT. Within a couple of months my blood glucose levels had returned to borderline diabetic.

At that point, rather than resume HIT, I decided to make myself the subject of another documentary in which I tested IF, intermittent fasting. As I describe in my book, *The Fast Diet*, on this regime I lost 20lb, most of it fat, and my blood glucose once more returned to normal.

These days I maintain my weight and improved glucose control through a combination of Intermittent Fasting and Fast Exercises.

The bad news was that, although I was able to push myself longer and harder on the exercise bike than I had on my previous visit and felt good about it, my aerobic fitness had not significantly improved. Despite sticking to the protocol, my heart and lungs were apparently in no better shape than they had been before I began doing HIT.

Although Jamie had warned me this might happen, it was still a nasty shock.

So why didn't HIT improve my aerobic fitness in the way that it had improved my insulin sensitivity? Why does it work better for some people than for others? The answer, as so often seems to be the case, lies in the genes.

## The genetics of exercise

As I wrote at the beginning of this chapter, one of the most widely accepted beliefs about exercise is that the more you do the fitter you become. Like the link between exercise and weight loss, it seems so self-evidently true, so in line with common sense, that it is madness to suggest otherwise. Perhaps you will never become an Olympic athlete or run the mile in less than 10 minutes, but if you train regularly then surely you must be making your heart and lungs stronger, adding years to your life. Sadly, life is not that fair.

'What we've known for quite some time now,' Jamie said, 'is that there's a huge variation in how people respond to an exercise regime and there's actually no guarantee that following any particular recipe will produce favourable results.'

There have, in fact, been a number of studies showing that the extent to which people respond to exercise varies wildly from person to person. In a recent study from Finland,[26] 175 untrained, middle-aged volunteers (89 men and 86 women) were asked to do a 21-week training course. The volunteers either did strength training (lifting weights) twice a week, endurance training twice a week or a workout which combined strength and endurance training 4 times a week.

The volunteers were carefully supervised to make sure they were actually doing the training and extensively tested before and after, measuring things like VO2 max and muscular strength.

The results were, to say the least, mixed. Some people's aerobic fitness improved by an impressive 42%, while others actually became less fit – their VO2 max dropped by 8%.

There was an even greater spread when it came to the strength exercises, with some people increasing their power output by 87% and others performing 12% worse at the end than they had at the beginning.

If this was the only study you might suspect that these were freakish results or that some of the volunteers were slacking. But there have been quite a number of studies that have come up with similar findings. The phenomenon has not been much commented on before because scientists tend to lump all data together and look for 'average' results. Anomalies get ignored, treated as outliers.

The implication of this and other studies, however, is that there is a huge range in people's responses to exercise – from super-responders at one end of the spectrum, those who will get a lot of benefit from doing regular exercise, to non-responders at the other, who are likely to get little.

## So how do you know whether you are a so-called super-responder or a non-responder?

The most reliable way to get an answer to this question would be to do what the volunteers did in the Finnish trial: get yourself measured and then put yourself through 21 weeks of hard training. That way you would find out which end of the spectrum you belong to. The other option might be to have a blood test.

When Jamie and his collaborators investigated the reasons for the variations in people's response to exercise, they discovered that when it comes to aerobic fitness much of the difference can be traced to the genetic code contained within just 11 genes. On the basis of this finding they developed a genetic test that they claim can accurately predict how well an individual will respond to exercise.

Before starting my HIT programme Jamie took a sample of my blood and sent it off to be DNA-tested. He didn't tell me the results until I'd done my 4 weeks of HIT.

After I had come back, been retested and expressed disappointment that my aerobic fitness had not improved in line with my expectations (from the studies, I was hoping for at least a 10% improvement), Jamie brought out the results of my genetic test. They were not good. Or rather, from his perspective, they were very good.

Of the more than 700 people they had tested at that time, my results were among the lowest. I had the fewest 'positive' versions of the genes that seem to promote improvements in VO2 max. As soon as he saw these results Jamie had been convinced that I would be a non-responder when it came to improving aerobic fitness. He was right.

As a human being I'm sure he would have been

delighted to give me better news, but as a scientist he was quietly pleased at the accuracy of his predictions.

I was naturally profoundly disappointed, but also not wholly surprised. I think, in my bones, I have always known that exercise doesn't do for me what it seems to do for a lot of other people.

That said, I don't believe that genes are destiny, so I take these sorts of tests with a pinch of salt. Jamie's test, I'm sure, is more accurate than most, but inevitably it's still not 100%.

There's no doubt that we are going to see a lot more genetic tests being sold in the future, tests which try to predict not only whether you are a responder/non-responder when it comes to aerobic fitness, but also whether exercise is likely to improve your glucose tolerance or whether you have the genes that will ensure that weight lifting will lead to bigger muscles.

A few of these gene tests will be useful, while others are likely to be of very low predictive value.

Some scientists hate the idea of these tests, not only because of the potential hype, but also because they fear that if they become widely available and people discover that they are non-responders they will simply give up all exercise.

I think this is unlikely to happen because even if you are a non-responder when it comes to one aspect of exercise, hopefully you are going to be a responder for another. I'm clearly never going to be a record-breaking long-distance runner but I am pleased that exercise has such a beneficial effect on my insulin. And, despite being something of an exercise-phobe, I have discovered that regular Fast Exercise makes me feel good and helps me keep the weight off.

Anyway, the upside to having a test which tells 20% of the population that they are non-responders is that the same tests will tell most people that they are responders and a lucky few (around 20% of the population) that if they take up exercise they are going to get enormous benefit. Peta, for example, was always likely to be a super-responder with an impressively large VO2 max (see page 173 for her score).

## Peta's DNA profile

Like Michael, I entered into the world of fitness DNA testing with some scepticism. As a lifelong exerciser what, I wondered, would the results reveal that I didn't already know?

Experience told me that I would probably be a responder. I've always found exercise not just easy but rewarding. While I knew I wasn't born with the 'fast twitch muscle fibres' that would make me a good sprinter, hockey player or jumper, and that I didn't have the genetic build that would allow me to bulk up with lots of weight training, I have always enjoyed endurance training such as long-distance running.

There are several companies that offer DNA testing. I tried two of the more established ones, with interesting results. The first suggested I was indeed a high aerobic responder, best suited to endurance-type activities – a conclusion which fits perfectly with my fitness background.

But when I sent a swab off to the second company they told me that my endurance potential was low and my abilities were much better suited to power and strength activities such as sprinting, weight training and sports such as netball and football – for none of which, I might add, I have ever displayed the remotest bit of enthusiasm or aptitude. It could be, of course, that I have hidden talents and have missed sporting opportunities as a result of not knowing my genetic weaknesses. But I don't think so.

Clearly, the development of DNA tests is in its infancy and they are not yet completely reliable – viz. my contradictory results. Still, if, as in Michael's case, they can help explain shortcomings and encourage you to focus your workouts more effectively, these tests certainly have a role to play. They have the potential to become a useful tool, helping us understand how individuals respond to exercise in starkly different ways.

# Is HIT safe?

With any form of exercise there is a risk that you will cause yourself some damage, particularly if you are not fit. The most common injuries are pulled muscles – which, as we all know, are easily incurred.

I have been to a few school sports days, particularly when my children were young, where the organisers have unwisely decided to include a 'Fathers' Race'. We fathers sheepishly volunteer, trying to look cool but secretly either dreading failure or hoping desperately to win. Some of the more competitive dads come in spiked training shoes; most of us come unprepared. We line up, our kids watching, keen not to disappoint. There is a shout, 'go', and we sprint off faster than is wise.

Ten strides in and at least one of the dads is down, as if shot, clutching a hamstring or possibly his groin. I know this situation, I speak from personal experience, I have been there, done it, lain screaming on the ground calling for ice.

While pulling a muscle is painful, it is certainly not fatal. The real fear is that if you are unfit and then begin to do vigorous exercise the unexpected shock will lead to a heart attack or stroke. And this fear is magnified 20-fold when people think about HIT. They imagine a sweaty, overweight man in Lycra with furred up arteries getting onto his bike and, wham, a few strokes in, his flabby overworked heart packs up, leaving behind a grieving family.

So is this fear justified? As you'll see in Chapter 3, 'Fast Exercise: the Workouts', we suggest that if you are unfit you should ease yourself into HIT. I would also always recommend that anyone who has any doubts about their health should have a medical check-up before starting any form of exercise.

One of the factors that could trigger a heart attack or stroke is a dramatic rise in blood pressure. This is more likely to happen if you are doing something like weight training than if you are doing aerobic exercise. Your heart rate rises quite dramatically while doing HIT and that could put strain on the heart, which is why it is important to build up the amount of HIT you do over a period of time, allowing your body time to adjust.

In my view, though, the most compelling reason for believing that HIT is safe, even in the elderly or unfit, is that it has been tested on precisely those people who are most at risk of having a heart attack: people who have previously had one.

## HIT and the heart: overturning accepted wisdom

When I was a medical student the accepted wisdom was that people who had had a heart attack and survived should take it easy. They were told to lie in bed, rest the heart, recover. Textbooks from the mid-1980s state unequivocally that 'reduced activity is critical in patients with heart failure'. This made perfect sense at the time – after all, if you'd had a near-fatal shock then surely rest was what was needed.

Then medical researchers did large-scale randomised trials and began to realise that this was not the best advice.

Trials like HF-ACTION, published in 2009,[27] showed that your chances of dying were significantly greater if you took to your bed. Common sense turned out to be wrong and now accepted wisdom has been turned on its head. These days doctors will advise you to mobilise as soon as possible, get back on your feet and get moving, often within days of your heart attack.

There has, therefore, been a paradigm shift, and I suspect that this shift will, in time, also embrace HIT. Over the last decade a number of trials have been carried out in different countries looking at the risks and benefits of HIT in those with heart disease, and HIT always comes out well.

In a Norwegian study,[28] researchers compared the risks of having a heart attack or stroke after doing HIT or moderate intensity training in a group of high-risk patients.

They took 4846 patients with coronary heart disease from rehabilitation centres and randomly allocated them either to moderate intensity training or to HIT. The patients who did moderate training, such as walking or jogging, put in a total of 129,456 hours of exercise. The HIT group did their exercise more intensely, but put in far fewer hours, a total of 46,364.

During a grand total of 175,820 hours of training in this high-risk group of patients there was one fatal heart attack. This was in the moderate training group. There were also two non-fatal heart attacks, in the HIT group.

The researchers' conclusion was that the risks, even in those with existing heart disease, of moderate or intense exercise are low, and that 'considering the significant cardiovascular adaptations associated with high intensity exercise, such exercise should be considered among patients with coronary heart disease'.

Similarly, in a review paper from 2012, 'High intensity interval training in cardiac rehabilitation', the authors looked at all the studies they could find that tested HIT in patients with coronary artery disease or heart failure. They concluded that 'HIT appears to be safe and better tolerated by patients than moderate intensity continuous exercise (MICE)'.

They go on to say that it is superior to standard exercise when it comes to producing improvements in heart function and quality of life.

Most recently a review paper from February 2013,[29] 'High intensity aerobic exercise in chronic heart failure', came to a similar conclusion: 'High intensity interval training is more effective than moderate intensity continuous exercise (MICE) for improving exercise capacity in patients with heart failure.'

Clearly, more research is required, but what I take from the studies done so far is that HIT – in fact any form of aerobic exercise – is more likely to cut your risk of having a heart attack or stroke than cause you to have one.

If you have any health concerns, see your doctor. Otherwise it's time to get your trainers on. In the next chapter, Peta will put you through your paces.

# FAST EXERCISE: THE
# WORKOUTS

The great thing about Fast Exercise is that it can be worked into a busy life with relative ease. It's less of a full-time commitment, more of an addition to the way you live. You can, if you really want, do Fast Exercise in your normal clothes, not even bothering to change into trainers, let alone gym kit. It's not something I do, but it is something Michael does. The fact it can be done in a suit or skirt without breaking sweat demonstrates how easily Fast workouts can be slotted into your day.

The other appealing thing about Fast Exercise is that it encompasses many different approaches, which is good because it's important to vary the way you exercise. Variety ensures you are kept on your toes, your body and mind never knowing what you are going to throw at them next.

Under the Fast Exercise umbrella we have included 2 types of exercise with very different purposes – Fast Fitness and Fast Strength. Both are extremely time-efficient. Within these 2 categories, we have also included a range of different plans. Find the one that suits you, but try also to vary them.

Fast Fitness is based on HIT, the aim being to boost your cardiovascular system and reduce your diabetes risk.

For good muscle tone and flexibility, however, we also suggest Fast Strength. These exercises strengthen the major muscle groups and rely on your body weight to achieve results. They can be done in a few minutes, without any special equipment, at home, at work, in a hotel room (all you need is a chair and tolerant neighbours) or while out for a run or walk (in which case you will need an empty park bench).

Depending on how long you want to spend warming up or cooling down, most Fast Fitness or Fast Strength exercises can be done in less than 10 minutes a day or just incorporated into what you are already doing.

The rule with HIT, or Fast Fitness, is to try and do 3 sessions a week, either as part of another exercise regime (i.e. add HIT to your run), as part of your commute (Michael often does it on his bike travelling home) or by itself. The temptation will probably be to do more. Don't. It won't make it more effective and the danger is, if you go crazy, you'll damage yourself.

When it comes to Fast Strength exercises, the rules are more flexible. Jamie Timmons works on his main muscle groups 3 times a week on days when he is not doing HIT. Michael likes to do them more often, up to 5 times a week. As do I, and I also vary my regime quite a bit – on nice days getting out to do a quick session in my local park (see the Park Workout on page 131).

Aim to split your time about 50-50 between Fast Fitness and Fast Strength, and you won't go far wrong. A typical weekly programme for the average exerciser, therefore, might comprise 2 days of Fast Fitness, 2 days of Fast Strength; and a typical week for those who are fitter and keener, say 3 days of Fast Fitness and 2 days of Fast Strength.

## Before you get going...

Warm-up and cool-down: how much, if any, is necessary? These are the bookends of any workout, the fitness components that promise to reduce injuries and fight fatigue. But are lengthy warm-ups and cool-downs as essential as every personal trainer would have us believe?

### The warm-up:
When it comes to HIT, most studies are based on a warm-up of 2-5 minutes of gentle, workout-specific activity (so, walking or running if you are sprinting, cycling if you are Fast Exercising on a bike, swimming if you are in the pool). Some researchers think you need less. There are no clear rules.

Michael warms up in just 1 minute for his cycle sessions, sometimes less. I prefer 5-10 minutes for running workouts. A warm-up should literally heat the body to increase blood flow, and loosen the muscles to ensure they are ready for activity. Warm muscles pull oxygen from the bloodstream more easily and trigger the chemical reactions needed to produce energy more efficiently. None of the workouts that are outlined on the pages that follow should be started without any preparation; how much is largely up to you.

## Stretching

It's widely believed that static stretching – the kind that involves holding a movement, such as bending over and touching your toes – makes your muscles more flexible, primes them for activity and reduces the chance of injury. That belief, widespread though it is, doesn't seem to be based on hard evidence. Indeed, the kind of stretches most of us think we should do before exercise – touching the toes or extending the hamstrings – have no obvious advantages and may be detrimental.

When Dr Ian Shrier, of the Centre for Epidemiology at the Jewish General Hospital in Montreal, reviewed the evidence on pre-workout stretching for *The Physician and Sports Medicine Journal* several years ago,[30] he found that stretching immediately before a gym session actually led to a reduction in muscle power. The effects were small and temporary, but significant enough for Shrier, a past president of the Canadian Academy of Sport Medicine, to recommend dropping stretches from warm-ups.

There is also the question of whether stretching reduces injuries. Most studies suggest it doesn't. A review article in *Sports Medicine*[31] makes the sensible point that if the sport you are doing involves a lot of stop-start (i.e. football) then you might get some benefit from stretching; but if you are running, jogging or swimming, there is strong evidence that stretching has 'no beneficial effect on injury prevention'.

If you want to stretch before you start, make it dynamic, with movements such as arm circling and side-stepping. Dynamic movements send a message from the brain to the muscles saying, 'We are ready to work out'. Static stretching, by contrast, triggers an inhibitory response in the brain. For sports like football, dynamic stretching might mean a bit of ball kicking and dribbling.

## The cool-down:

Much less research has been conducted on the value of the cool-down and the research that has been done has produced little evidence either way. After a burst of intense exercise it is best not to stop moving entirely. When you work out really hard, the heart has to pump much faster, and blood vessels expand, leading to greater blood flow to the legs and feet. If you stop too suddenly, blood can start to pool in the lower limbs, causing dizziness.

Michael gets his HIT mainly from cycling and he spends about a minute doing gentle cycling after a fierce burst to allow his blood pressure and heart rate to return to normal. I, on the other hand, like to spend at least 5 minutes after a Fast workout doing the same activity at a slower pace. I find it brings everything back to equilibrium.

## The dreaded DOMS (Delayed Onset Muscle Soreness):

Another popular myth is that cool-down stretches will stop your muscles from becoming sore by flushing out lactic acid, one of the so-called waste products of exercise. Some gym instructors will tell you that it is the build-up of lactic acid that makes your muscles tired. This is nonsense.

Yes, strenuous exercise will lead to greater production of lactic acid but the reason this happens is because lactate is needed as a fuel. Without it you wouldn't be able to push yourself as hard as you do.

The soreness you get after exercise isn't caused by a build up of lactic acid, but by minor damage to muscle fibres, and stretching will have no effect on that. The only real remedy is rest.

In an Australian study, in which volunteers were asked to walk backwards on a treadmill for half an hour to induce calf-muscle stiffness,[32] researchers found that doing a warm-up made a small difference to perceived muscle soreness 2 days later but a 10-minute cool-down made no difference. Personally, I like to stretch at the end of the day. It helps me to relax and to unknot the tensions of the day. But find what works for you.

## Painkillers

A word of warning. You might be tempted to take anti-inflammatory agents like aspirin or ibuprofen before doing exercise to reduce muscle soreness afterwards. Don't. Numerous studies have shown that they won't reduce muscle soreness and that they can cause bleeding in the stomach and gastrointestinal leakage, bacteria getting out of your gut and into your blood.

## And finally, before you start: keeping track

We recommend you keep track of your progress in an exercise diary. The kinds of measurements you might record once a month or so could include:

- Strength – how many press-ups can you comfortably do?
- Resting heart rate
- Weight and waist measurement
- Your aerobic fitness, as measured by your VO2 max
- Your glucose tolerance

To find out how to do these, see the section on measuring the impact of exercise at the back of the book.

There are all sorts of activities that will enable you to get the intensity required for Fast Fitness. The following 6 are ordered according to the likely level of benefit revealed by research, but also according to our personal preference. Cycling is first because it is how most HIT studies have been done so far, and it's Michael's favourite (though he's partial to stair-running, too). Running comes next because it is a popular form of exercise, good for HIT, and it is my preferred way; cross-training is Jamie Timmons' favourite, also a good all-round form of training for those who prefer to work out in a gym. Of the rest, I would say that they are all good forms of exercise in themselves, but less is known about their particular suitability for HIT – and be careful with rowing, which has the potential to cause injury with poor technique.

## Cycling

Indoor cycling is a good way of getting HIT because a modern indoor bike lets you add resistance, changing the intensity of the ride. It also enables you to continue exercising when it's cold, wet and dark outside. And, unlike some other forms of exercise, it is less

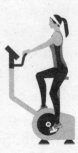

prone to cause injuries. Most of the academic studies on HIT have involved volunteers using special indoor stationary bikes because they are well suited to laboratory studies. However, many people prefer the fresh air and unpredictable terrain they encounter outside. On a road or mountain bike the exercise intensity can be altered by switching to a higher gear and by cycling hard uphill. Wind can also add resistance, making an outdoor cycle more intense.

## Running

Running (or jogging) requires no special equipment, other than a pair of trainers, a T-shirt and some shorts. It can be done almost anywhere and offers clear health benefits in its own right.

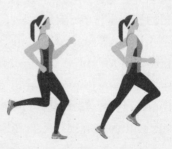

To make a normal run into HIT you will have to inject intensity into your workout, which means you need to throw in a few sprints, preferably up a hill. By pushing your body on an incline you are working your muscles much harder than when you run on the flat. A hill should be challenging but not so steep that you can't run up it fast. If you are not especially fit, build up to this gradually.

Start by trying to run flat out up a hill for 10 seconds. As you get fitter, build slowly up to, say, 30 seconds. After running up a hill you should avoid jogging back down; walk down instead.

Use natural markers (trees, lampposts) to establish distances, or a stopwatch to time your sprints. Try to vary the terrain on which you run – grass, dirt trails, running tracks and pavements are all suitable.

Running well uphill requires rhythm: shorten your stride slightly compared to when you are running on the flat and aim to keep your leg turnover constant. Don't lean forward from the waist or back – your head, shoulders and back should form a straight line over your feet.

## Running on a treadmill

There are two kinds of runner: those who like treadmills and those who don't. Personally, I can't see the appeal of the hamster-wheel confinement of a mechanical running belt, but many people find the treadmill reassuringly familiar. Nothing ever changes – no wind, no rain, no traffic – so they know exactly what to expect.

When it comes to performing HIT on a treadmill, the major downside is having to deal with the mechanics. Switching speeds between the desired intensity for HIT and recovery can be tricky and is almost never instant. Studies have also shown that indoor running burns about 5% fewer calories than running outdoors, partly because of the lack of wind resistance and partly because the treadmill's motorised belt propels you slightly. For these reasons, it's advisable to crank up the gradient in order to make sure you are working hard enough. Research at the University of Brighton suggests treadmill users who want to achieve the same workload intensity as running on flat terrain outdoors need to set the machine at a permanent 1% incline.

## Stair-running

If you have access to several flights of stairs, either at work or at home, they constitute a terrific HIT circuit. The American Lung Foundation says that stair-running provides the same benefits as conventional running in half the time, because you are constantly working against gravity. Stair-running is fairly low-impact on the knees and feet and is one of the best activities for bottom- and leg-toning. Make sure you use good technique: don't

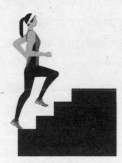

hunch your back or twist your head, and bend your arms at right angles to provide power as they pump. Make sure that your whole foot lands on each step, to avoid straining the Achilles tendon – and walk (don't run) back downstairs during recovery periods. Or take the lift.

## Cross-training

With a cross-trainer you can work lots of different muscles in a short period of time. Set it on the highest incline and resistance. Gently move your arms and legs for 1 minute to loosen up. Then pick up the tempo, aiming to give a maximum effort (high tempo) for about 30 seconds, before slowing down.

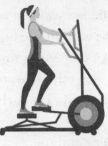

## Swimming

It is the natural resistance of water that makes swimming physically challenging, and the faster you try to swim, the harder you are going to have to

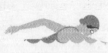

work. Swimming uses a lot of muscles but it is important to occasionally vary the strokes. Rather than judging things by time it may be easier to judge by distance. A 25-metre length at full pelt is comparable to sprinting for around 30-40 seconds.

## Rowing

An indoor rowing machine will, like a cross-trainer, work

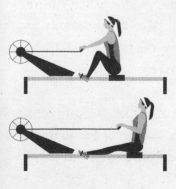

the entire body and be extremely challenging, but it is one of those pieces of equipment you need to be wary of as you can hurt yourself quite badly if you don't know what you are doing. Good technique is crucial. Start each stroke by pushing with the legs, not pulling with the arms, and keep your wrists in line with the handle so that the pulley wire is parallel to the floor. Make sure your back is straight, not rounded, to increase the power of each stroke and reduce the pressure on your lower back.

## Skipping

Skipping, like running, is convenient. However, it's quite hard to involve lots of muscle groups and achieve the necessary intensity. Avoid buying traditional woven ropes 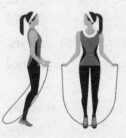 as these are heavy (even more so when wet) and slow to turn. Ball bearings and jump counters also add unnecessary weight and make ropes more cumbersome. Your best bet is a lightweight, flexible plastic or leather gymnastic 'speed' rope. Knees and ankles should be flexed but your torso kept straight when jumping. Arms should be at your side with the rope turning from the wrists and forearms.

## The workouts

In the next few pages, I outline a variety of Fast Fitness workouts. Between us Michael and I have tried and tested every variation on the theme. We each have our favourites among the suggestions below. And we each have those that we feel are bringing benefit even if we don't always relish the prospect of completing them. Just remember: the discomfort (and there should be an element of puffing, panting, muscle soreness and all-over fatigue) is temporary. In less than the time it takes to drive to the gym it will all be over.

The following workouts should ideally be done 2-3 times a week. We have ordered them roughly in terms of the amount of time you spend doing the intense part of the exercise. The total amount of time you actually spend on each workout will depend on a number of factors, including how long you choose to warm up and cool down.

The actual intensity of the exercise is up to you; wearing a heart-rate monitor will give you an indication of how hard you are pushing yourself, but the important thing is to start slowly and build up gradually so your body has time to adapt. Don't overdo it on the first day.

## The Bare Minimum

*40 seconds' hard exercise (2 x 20 seconds)*
*Total – 4-6 minutes, including recovery*

Unbelievably, there is evidence that just 40 seconds of

intense activity can make a difference. In 2011 Dr Niels Vollaard and colleagues at Bath University did a study[33] in which they asked 15 healthy but sedentary young men and women to try something they called REHIT (reduced exertion high intensity training) for 6 weeks.

He started them off in the first week with a couple of minutes of gentle cycling, then one 10-second burst of intense cycling followed by a couple of minutes of cool-down. In weeks 2 and 3, each exercise session consisted of a warm-up, 15 seconds of all-out sprinting, a couple of minutes of recovery, another 15 seconds of all-out sprinting, then the gentle cool-down.

For the final 3 weeks they cranked it up so each exercise session consisted of two 20-second flat-out sprints separated by a couple of minutes of recovery.

Despite the fact that over the 6 weeks the volunteers had done less than 10 minutes of hard exercise, both the men and the women showed significant improvements in their aerobic fitness (VO2 max up 15% and 12% respectively). When it came to insulin sensitivity, there was a gender difference: the men's improved by 28% while the women's did not improve.

Niels is currently carrying out further studies to see if this gender difference is real and also to see if people with metabolic syndrome and diabetes get similar improvements.

He is also keen, at some point, to see if a single burst of 20 seconds done 3 times a week makes a measurable difference. If you are only doing a few bursts 20 seconds seems to be the minimum time for a burst that will make a difference.

The basic principle here is to push yourself in 2 brief 20-second bursts. The most obvious activity to choose is cycling, since that was what they did in the trials; if you are doing it indoors, you will need an exercise bike with variable resistance on which you can crank up the intensity mechnically; and, if cycling outside, you will need to find a hill, preferably quite a steep one, and use gravity to increase your workload. But in principle, any of the activities above will work fine. In the case of running, you will need to find some way of cranking up the resistance for your 20-second spurts – either mechanically, on a treadmill in the gym, or by using a hill if you are outside.

- Start off with a couple of minutes of gentle pedalling/running/swimming.

- When you feel ready, speed up and work your body as hard as you can for 20 seconds, before slowing down.

- Repeat the sprint after you've had a couple of minutes of gentle pedalling/jogging/walking to recover. Recovery time is important.

In total the Bare Minimum should take less than 10

minutes. Michael likes to do it on an exercise bike (see box below) and, now that he's more used to it, he does it in less than 4 minutes by minimising warm-up and cool-down and by cutting his gentle pedalling to about a minute.

If you are very unfit or have never tried HIT before, it may be worth slowly building up the sprints from 2 x 10 seconds to 2 x 20 seconds. Once you have mastered 2 x 20 seconds you may want to add on another 20-second sprint which, along with the recom-mended recovery period, will add another couple of minutes to your regime.

## How Michael does it

1. Put the kettle on.
2. Get on the exercise bike and do a couple of minutes of gentle cycling, against limited resistance. You should just about notice the effort in your thighs.
3. After about 2 minutes begin pedalling fast, then swiftly crank up the resistance.
4. The amount of resistance you select will depend on your current strength and fitness. It should be high enough that after 15 seconds of sprinting your thighs begin to burn and the speed at which you are pedalling slows, simply because your muscles are fatigued and you cannot

keep going at that pace.

5. If, after 15 seconds, you can still keep going at the same pace then the resistance you've chosen is not quite high enough. It mustn't, however, be so high that you grind to a complete halt. It's a matter of experimenting. What you'll find is that as you get fitter the amount of resistance you can cope with increases. It is important that you keep increasing the resistance to ensure each 20-second workout involves maximum effort.

6. After your first burst of fast sprinting, drop the resistance and do a couple of minutes of gentle pedalling to catch your breath and let your muscles recharge.

7. Then, when you feel ready, do another 20-second burst.

8. Relax! Its over! Finish with a couple of minutes of gentle cycling to allow your heart rate and blood pressure to return to normal before stepping off the bike and having a cup of tea.

## How Peta gets her 20-second HIT while running

The Bare Minimum workout doesn't have to be a stand-alone session. I prefer to weave it into a slightly longer run or walk of 15-20 minutes rather than head to the park for just 40 seconds of exercise. My approach is to run at a moderate pace for 5-10 minutes and then perform the lung-burning 20-second flat-out burst. I then jog for another 3-4 minutes before doing the second sprint and finish with a 5-minute gentle run. Those short bursts are tougher than you might think. If you do them properly with pumping arms and fast leg speed, you will feel your thighs burn and your heart rate soar after each one – which is a positive thing. Personally, I like to do the sprints around the edge of a football or cricket pitch so that I can try to get a bit further each time I do it. But fit them in when and where you can – even on the walk to school or work.

## How to do the Bare Minimum at work

Fast Exercise can be done at work, whether your employer provides a gym or not, as long as you work somewhere with at least 4 flights of stairs.

You can do this regime in a suit, but if you wear high heels you will need to replace them with more sensible flat rubber-soled shoes.

First find a quiet stairwell in a building with at least 4 full floors. If you are unfit, you may want to spend a few weeks walking up the 4 flights before attempting anything more adventurous.

When you feel up to it, try bounding up the stairs for 20 seconds. And I mean *bounding*. If you are a beginner, this should be long enough to make you breathe heavily and to feel the build-up of fatigue in your thighs. As you get fitter you will find that you need to run for longer, up more stairs, to get the same feeling.

Ideally take the lift down to where you started, or in a tall building just pause for 1-2 mins to catch your breath before bounding up another few floors.

## The 30-Second Sprinter

*2 minutes' hard exercise*
*Total – 16 minutes, including 14 minutes' recovery*

This is similar to the 20-second sprints that we have just described, except that you will need a longer recovery period between sprints because going from 20 seconds to 30 seconds of all-out sprinting is much more demanding.

If you are not used to HIT, you should start gradually, preferably by working your way through a 20-second regime first, then trying 2 x 30 seconds and building up from there.

Make time to do a couple of minutes of warm-up and ensure you are mentally ready before starting your first sprint. Between each sprint pedal gently for 3-4 minutes to recover (you will need it).

This regime is based on the original HIT studies, which were done in Canada and were called SIT (sprint interval training). The Canadians found that doing four 30-second sprints (interspersed with a few minutes of recovery) 3 times a week led to similar improvements in fitness as running or cycling at a steady speed for many hours a week.[34]

**30-second sprint/bike:** 4 x 30-second sprints on a bike. Make time to do a couple of minutes warm up before starting your first sprint. Between each sprint take 3-4 minutes to recover by pedalling at a gentle pace (you will need it). Then take at least 2 minutes to cool down.

**30-second sprint/run:** 4 x 30-second running sprints up a hill. Warm up by running at a gentle pace to your chosen hill. Then sprint for 30 seconds up the hill; walk down or around for a few minutes, then do it again. And again. And again. Finish by jogging slowly home. Stretch if you like.

**30-second sprint/swim:** If you like swimming, do the first few lengths at a gentle pace. When you are ready, try swimming 25 metres flat out (or count to 30 in your head). Take a bit of a breather, then continue gently swimming a couple more lengths. Then do another sprint. Repeat 4 times. Finish with a very gentle couple of lengths.

# The 60-Second Workout

*2½ minutes' hard exercise*
*Total – 10-11 minutes, including 8 minutes' recovery*

This is one of my favourite approaches and a format I have used for many years. It's very simple: the basic principle is to alternate 60-second bursts of activity with 90-second recovery periods – i.e. 1 minute on, 1½ minutes off. It's wonderfully flexible: it can be done with any of the activities listed above, i.e. cycling, running, swimming, and can be scaled down or up according to what you require.

You might think that 60 seconds of HIT has to be tougher than 30 seconds, but this version is not. The 60-second workout evolved out of work done by the sports science team at McMaster University when they were trying to find an effective but 'gentler' version of the challenging 30-Second Sprinter. The key difference is that you don't push yourself quite as hard. Instead of going flat out, you exercise for a minute at about 90% of your best effort, aiming to push your heart rate up to around 80% of HR max (see section on measuring the impact of exercise at the back of the book) by the end of the first minute (to find out your HR max, see the reference section at the back).

In the original studies they asked the volunteers to do 10 x 1-minute bursts of HIT with 90 seconds recovery in between each burst. This is what I do. More recently researchers from Metapredict (a group of exercise academics) have begun testing a less demanding variant, involving a maximum of 5 x 60-second bursts alternated with 90-second recovery periods.

The less fit should definitely start with 3 bursts; if you are super-keen, and really want to push the boat out, you can do the full 10 (this is effectively the Roger Bannister version, and particularly beneficial if you are preparing for an endurance event). Our recommendation, if you are basically quite fit, is that you aim for a steady 5. So:

- 2 minutes of warm-up.

- 5 x 60-second bursts of activity, with 90 seconds' recovery between each burst.

- 1 minute of cool-down.

## The Fat Burner

*8 minutes' hard exercise*
*Total – 20 minutes, including 12 minutes' recovery*

This workout involves a repetitive cycle of 8 seconds of intense activity alternated with 12 seconds of recovery, and is only really suitable for an exercise bike. It is based on two key Australian studies by Stephen Boutcher,[35] which showed that HIT could lead to significant fat loss.

After a brief warm-up, you cycle hard against resistance for 8 seconds, then gently for 12, then hard against resistance again for 8 seconds and gently for 12, and so on.

To begin with, you maintain this pattern for about 5 minutes. The aim, as you get fitter, is to build up to 15 or even 20 minutes. The resistance stays constant throughout the 20 minutes, high enough so it feels strenuous. Gradually build up resistance over the first few weeks.

## The 4-Minute Pelter

*Total – 4 minutes' hard exercise*

This is different because, instead of exerting yourself in intervals, you are doing it all in one go. Norwegian researchers found that a single 4-minute burst of running/jogging/walking on a treadmill at a hard pace done 3 times a week was enough to boost the health and fitness of previously sedentary middle-aged men significantly. At the end of their 10-week trial the men had improved their aerobic capacity by 10% or more, lost a couple of pounds of fat, lowered their blood pressure and had better blood sugar control.[36]

**4-minute pelter/bike:** After a warm-up, do 4 minutes of hard cycling at around 90% of maximal effort.

**4-minute pelter/run:** After a warm-up, do one 4-minute run at 90% of your maximum pace (this will leave you tired and breathless. You should definitely not be chatting). An alternative is to see how far you can run in 4 minutes – and try to better it next time. Do it in the local park, using markers such as trees or posts. Or try it on an athletics track.

**4-minute pelter/stair sprint:** Run hard up a flight of stairs and walk back down the same flight, covering as many 'fast' flights as possible in 4 minutes. As you get fitter, try to increase the number of flights you can manage in the time-span. You should be able to manage about 10 flights.

**4-minute pelter/walk:** The researchers recommend a brisk 4-minute walk uphill at an 8-10% gradient (this is quite steep), perhaps to or from work.

# Fast Walking

This is a great staple, which can be built easily into your day – your walk to work, to and from the local shops – and is surprisingly effective. Walking up a hill, fast enough to get your pulse racing, is ideal but it can also be done on the flat. Like other forms of Fast activity, Fast Walking (where you alternate fast with slow) seems to have more impact than ordinary low intensity strolling. The studies I've seen (see page 162) show that it leads to more fat loss, improved fitness and glucose control. The studies are based on walking fast in 3-minute bursts. If you're not fit, then aim for something more modest, like 1-2 minutes.

- Begin by walking at a normal pace, just to warm up.

- When you are ready, pick up the pace. On the RPF (rated perceived exertion) scale where 1 is light and 10 is very hard, you should be aiming at 6-7 – it should be hard, but you should be able to keep going. Then slow down and give yourself at least 3 minutes of slower walking to recover.

- Repeat a couple of times.

- Start off by trying a 20-minute Fast Walk a couple

of times a week. As you get fitter, increase the length of the walk and the number of times you put in a Fast burst.

## FAST STRENGTH – WORKING WITH YOUR BODYWEIGHT

For maximum health gains, you need to exercise not only your heart and lungs but also other major muscle groups. Fast Strength is a form of circuit training, except it can be done at home without special equipment and it is best done fast. The idea is to exercise as many major muscle groups as possible, and to alternate between activities in such a way as to give the ones not being worked a bit of a rest. So, if you are doing push-ups (working the upper body), you should follow these with an activity that works the core (say, abdominal crunches) or the legs (squats).

Similarly, if you've just done a workout that produces a big increase in heart rate, such as jumping jacks, the next exercise should be one that is more sedate, such as a wall-sit.

To pack it all into as little time as possible and to maximise metabolic impact you should do as many repeats of each exercise as you can manage in 30 seconds and take just 10 seconds' rest between each.

The Fast Strength approach is based on a paper in the *American College of Sports Medicine's Health & Fitness Journal*[37] and is now one of Michael's favourite regimes.

This approach is designed to combine aerobic and resistance training and it can, as the song says, be done any time, anywhere. Although you should start by doing one 7-minute session twice a week, as you get fitter you may want to fit in a few more sessions, and also vary the exercises.

There is nothing new about the exercises that are recommended in the paper, just the way the combinations are put together.

A note of caution: if you have elevated blood pressure (hypertension), it is best to avoid isometric exercises like the wall-sit, the side-plank and the plank.

Suggested exercises:

## Jumping jacks

Stand with your hands by your sides. In one movement, jump up, spreading your legs apart as you raise your arms and over your head. You should land with your arms over your head and your feet more than hip-width apart. Jump up again and in one movement, bring your legs together and your arms back to your sides. You have just done one jumping jack. Keep going for 30 seconds.

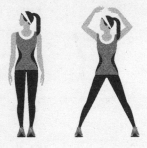

## Press-ups

Lie face down with the palms of your hands directly beneath your shoulders and the balls of your feet touching 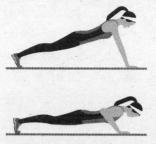 the ground. Keep your body straight – your head in line with your back – and raise yourself up using your arms. Lower your torso to the ground until your elbows form a 90-degree angle and then push up again. If you find this too hard, perform the exercise with your knees on the ground until you are strong enough to do the full thing. Record how many you can do in 30 seconds.

---

## Wall-sit

Start with your back against a wall with your feet shoulder-width apart and positioned about 2 feet from the wall. 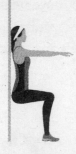 Slowly slide your back down the wall until your thighs are parallel with the ground. Adjust your feet if you need to so that your knees are directly above your ankles (rather than over your toes). Don't arch your back. Hold this position, if you can, for 30 seconds.

---

## Abdominal crunches

Lie on your back with your knees bent and feet flat on the floor and your hands positioned by your sides (or lightly at the sides of your head). Curl up your upper body without lifting your lower back off the floor.

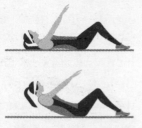

Make sure your chin is tucked in towards your chest. When your shoulders and upper back are lifted off the floor, curl back down. Again, it's 30 seconds.

---

## Step-ups on a chair

Use a bench or sturdy chair with a seat that is at a comfortable height to step onto. Place one foot on the

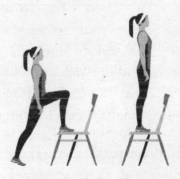

'step', making sure your whole foot is in contact with the surface. Push your body weight up, driving your weight through your heel and breathing out as you do this, until you are standing on top of the step with both feet. Step back and down, one leg at a time until you are standing with both feet flat on the floor again. Repeat with the opposite leg leading. Step-ups should be performed with care but at a brisk pace, for – you guessed it – 30 seconds.

## Squats

Stand with feet shoulder-width apart and hands placed lightly on opposite shoulders. Bend from the hips, keeping the weight in your heels. Make sure your back is straight. Keep bending until your legs are at a 90-degree angle – imagine you are preparing to sit in a chair. Push back up without bending your back.

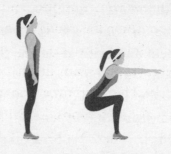

## Tricep dips

Stand with your back to a bench or chair; place your palms on the seat behind you, bending your knees at right angles, hips straight. Bend your elbows to 90 degrees to lower your body (so that your bottom descends halfway to the floor). Push yourself back up using only your arms.

## Plank

Lie on the floor and then raise yourself onto your forearms and toes so that your body forms a straight line from head to toe. Make sure your mid-section doesn't rise or drop.

Squeeze your buttocks and hold
the position for as long as possible.
Remember, this exercise should
never cause pain in the lower
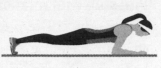
back. The first time you try this you probably won't
manage 30 seconds. Do what you can.

## High-knee running
Stand tall and begin jogging either on the spot or forward.
Without leaning back, drive through the balls of your feet
and try to bring your knees close
to chest level. Keep your hands
relaxed, elbows bent and
shoulders down, and swing your
arms back and forth to help you
keep going. Again, 30 seconds of
this is hard work. Start slow.

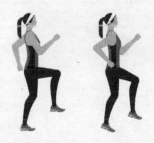

## Lunge
Stand with your back straight and
feet shoulder-width apart. Step
forward with one leg, bending both
knees to 90 degrees and keeping your
upper body straight. Pull back to the
starting position and repeat, putting
the other leg forward.

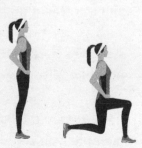

## Press-up with rotation

Assume the classic press-up position (above), but as you straighten your arms in the upward move, rotate your body so that your right arm extends overhead. Your arms and torso should form a 'T'. Return to the starting position, lower yourself by bending your elbows, then push up and rotate till your left hand points towards the ceiling.

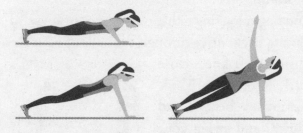

## Side-plank

Lie on your side and raise your body so that your weight is supported by your lower forearm and feet. Maintain a diagonal line 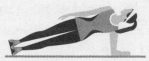 with your body, keeping your hips off the floor. Make sure your neck and back are straight. Hold for as long as possible.

These are the basics. But there are lots of variants. For example, you could try a:

★ **Plank with leg raise**: Lie face down with your

elbows on the ground; elevate your body, keeping your weight distributed between your forearms and feet. Your elbows should be bent at a 90-degree angle. Keep your back straight with your hips raised off the floor. Squeeze your torso tight, slowly lifting one foot 6-8 inches off the ground and hold the position for a few seconds. Lower your leg back to the starting position.

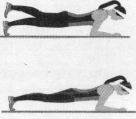

★ **Side-plank with reach-around**: Lie on your side and elevate your body, supporting your weight between your forearm and feet. Keep your body straight with your hips off the floor; your neck and back should stay straight. Raise your upper arm straight above you so that it's perpendicular to the floor. Reach under and behind your torso with that hand, then lift your arm back up to the starting position.

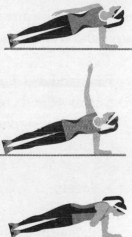

★ **Reverse curl**: as an alternative to the plank, lie on your back, with your hands by your sides, your feet up and your thighs perpendicular to the floor. They should not go lower than this for the entire movement. Using your lower abs, roll your pelvis to raise your hips off the floor. Your legs will now be at a 45-degree angle to the floor. Return slowly to the start position.

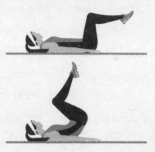

### Even Faster HIT

There are all sorts of ways you can mix up these particular exercises. The following circuits can all be done in just 4 minutes. Make sure you include variety so that your legs, arms and trunk muscles are all worked.

**Fast ladder:** Choose 4 exercises from either of the lists above and do them 10 times each, then 9 times, then 8 times – until you perform just one repetition of each. My preferred routine is:

- Squats
- Lunges
- 10-metre sprint shuttle runs (i.e. back-to-back sprints). Only practical if you are outside.
- Tricep dips

**Fast max-reps:** Choose 3 of the body-weight (Fast Strength) exercises listed above, do each one 10 times. Move as fast as you possibly can to get through as many rounds as possible in 4 minutes.

## The Park Workout

It might sound an odd admission for a fitness writer, but I'm no fan of gyms. I find the gym environment sterile and far from motivational; I feel self-conscious surrounded by mirrors and super-toned workout fanatics. Gym classes, too, leave me exasperated with their choreographed content and repetition. But most of all I miss being outdoors.

Exercise outside and your skin is kissed by the breeze. There is exposure to real, natural daylight that has untold benefits for mind and body – boosting your mood and vitamin D stores. Numerous studies have shown that outdoor or 'green' exercise improves not only our daily mood but our general mental health. Researchers at the University of Essex showed that just 5 minutes of workouts in the park enhanced subjects' mental wellbeing, while other studies have shown that people who have exerted themselves outside have lower blood levels of cortisol, a hormone related to stress, than those who have exercised inside.

More than anything else, perhaps, there is an element

of unpredictability that not only prevents you from getting bored, but actually helps you work harder. Studies have shown that exercising outdoors on undulating ground and changing surfaces, often with wind for added resistance, uses far more energy than slapping the soles of your trainers on the conveyor belt of a treadmill.

Of course, Fast Exercise is perfectly suited to be performed indoors or out, but for something different I like to throw the odd park circuit into the mix. Some of the bench exercises below are the brainchild of sports scientist Steve Mellor. Others are exercises I myself have found to be effective over the years. So, find a tree, a path or a park bench and off you go.

Perform 10 repetitions of 2-4 of the exercises below, alternating them for a total of 3-6 minutes. Move as fast as you possibly can, and try and get through as many rounds as possible of the exercises in the time.

## Bear crawl

Put on some old clothes and head for the park. Start on all fours and begin moving along the ground as quickly as you can. Add variations – move the arm and leg from the

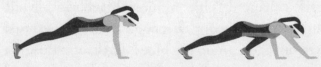

same side of your body at the same time, or move the opposite arm and foot. Keep your hips straight and low at first (as if stalking something in a bush) and then change to a high-level crawl. Crawl for 10 seconds.

## Log haul

This is fine, again, if you don't mind getting dirty, and should only be performed with a log or rock that is not so

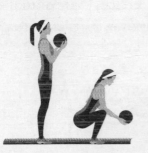

heavy that it is a strain to lift it. Squat down from the knees (keeping your back straight) to pick up the item and lift it, preferably to shoulder level. If it's too heavy, carry it with your arms straight, keeping good spinal alignment. Carry it a distance of 10 metres, aiming to move as quickly as possible.

## Deep squat

Stand with your feet wider than hip-width apart and your back straight. Bend your knees to drop down into as deep

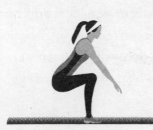

a squat as possible with your buttocks aiming for the ground. The position should feel relaxed and you should keep your heels on the ground. Allow your arms to hang in front of your body and keep your head in line with your spine. If you find this too difficult at first, try holding onto a bench or tree for support. Hold the position for 15 seconds.

## Mountain climber

Facing a bench, place your hands on the edge of the seat and extend your legs behind you in a press-up position with head, back and feet in a straight line. Drive one knee up in between the arms then drive the foot back down

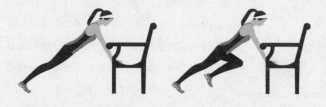

into the start position and quickly change legs. Only one foot should be on the floor at any one time – aim to mimic a sprinting style.

## Bench push-up

Assume a plank position by placing your hands on the front edge of a bench, your body in a straight line, so that your weight is supported on the balls of your feet and by your elbows (bent to 90 degrees). Don't allow your back to arch, or your hips to drop. Push up until your arms are straight; then lower them back down so that both elbows are bent at 90 degrees. Repeat.

## Bench get-up

Facing a bench, place your hands on the edge of the seat and extend your legs behind you in a press-up position with head, back and feet in a straight line. Step your right leg forward in line with the right hand. Do not allow the

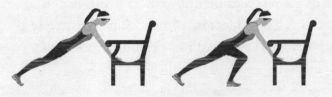

foot to come across the body. Push through right heel and stand up. Step back to start position and repeat on the other leg.

---

## Squat thrust push-up

Place your hands on the seat of a bench and assume a press-up position with your head, back and feet forming a straight line. Bend your elbows and then straighten

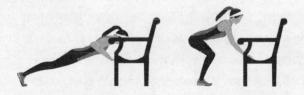

them to raise your body. Jump towards the bench and back to the start position, keeping your hands on the bench throughout.

# Michael's perspective

I first started building Fast Strength exercises into my regime when I came across the study, 'High Intensity Circuit Training using Body Weight' in the online version of the *American College of Sports Medicine's Health & Fitness Journal* in early 2013. As they point out at the beginning of the article, 'For exercise strategies to be practical and applicable to the time-constrained client, they must be safe, effective and efficient. As many of our clients travel frequently, the program also must be able to be performed anywhere, without special equipment.' They go on to state, citing a number of studies, 'that the combination of aerobic and resistance training in a high intensity, limited-rest design can deliver numerous health benefits in much less time than traditional programs'.

I travel quite a bit and have spent more evenings than I care to remember in foreign hotels. When I first read the article I was already practising HIT. But though I was doing aerobic training I was not doing anything about body strength. So I started straight away.

I found the exercises surprisingly easy to do, though when I am in a hotel I tend to skip the knee-high running as it seems rather unfair on anyone in the floor below who is trying to sleep.

I also discovered, on a recent trip to Australia,

where I met up with some old friends from medical school, a variant called 'The Park Bench Workout' — which is similar to the one proposed by Peta here.

As well as many of the exercises listed above, the Australian Park Bench Workout included one real killer, the Dip and Kick. It starts off like the triceps dip, but rapidly gets worse. You start with your hands behind you on the bench, your elbows bent at 90 degrees and your bottom a few inches off the ground. Then, instead of straightening, you have to kick out like a Russian Cossack, doing as many kicks as you can in 30 seconds.

I never really mastered this particular exercise, but on the whole Fast Strength workouts have done wonders for my fitness levels. I can now do 35 press-ups in 30 seconds and 20 squats without falling over. I have rediscovered abdominal muscles that I have not seen for years. Not yet a 6-pack, but getting there.

I also recently discovered, while doing press-ups at home, a pile of semi-empty pizza boxes under our bed. I'm now wondering which of the kids left them there.

## What happens when you hit a plateau?

As with all exercise programmes, there will come a time

when your body adapts to the training load that you are applying and will not respond as well as it did a few weeks previously. This is known as a fitness plateau – and we all hit them from time to time. It's at this point that you need to make tweaks to your regime, to raise your workouts to the next level so that your body begins to respond again.

This does not necessarily mean that you have to increase the duration of your session (although you can try one of the longer or shorter Fast workouts for variety). Progression can be achieved by increasing the intensity or speed of your 'efforts', by attempting to complete more moves in an allotted time or by shortening recovery time so that you can attempt a greater number of 'bursts'.

Forget the fable about the tortoise and the hare. When it comes to Fast Exercise it really is a case of short bursts of applied effort. In the next chapter I look at how to make Fast Exercise part of your daily life.

# FAST EXERCISE IN PRACTICE

Over the years I've changed the way I exercise to suit my lifestyle. In my teens and twenties I devoted many hours a day to improving my running times and performances. But now, as a working mum with an 8-year-old son, my day gets gobbled up with play-dates, football and rugby matches. I still crave to be outside, breathing in the fresh air of the Chilterns countryside where I live. But I no longer have the time – or desire – to do lengthy workouts. And I've found that short, sharp bursts of HIT sessions suit me perfectly.

## When to exercise

The real appeal of Fast Exercise is that it can slip easily into your day. Even if you are time crunched, you can always find a few minutes to devote to this kind of condensed workout. It is better, however, that you don't just 'fit it in when you can'. If you commit to a regular time you are more likely to keep your regime going.

So is there any evidence that exercising at any particular time of the day is more beneficial?

If you are interested in performance, then late afternoon or early evening may be a better time to work out. Researchers at Liverpool John Moores University found that when people were asked to perform the same workout at different times of the day (5am, 11am, 5pm and 11pm), they felt they were working hardest first thing – though this wasn't necessarily the case. Top swimmers have been shown to suffer a 10% drop in performance during morning training sessions.

Why? Well, your body temperature is lowest first thing in the morning. It then steadily rises by about 1 degree Celsius till it reaches a peak around midday. It stays quite high till about 7pm, when it starts to fall.

Being slightly more revved up with warmer muscles may contribute to an improvement in performance. It may also reduce the risk of injury. On this basis exercising any time between midday and 7pm is good. Much later and it may disturb your sleep.

So is the afternoon best? Not necessarily. Sports scientists at Glasgow University say that, while morning exercise may feel harder for some people, it can be a great mood-booster, setting you up mentally for the day. Their research, published in the journal *Appetite*,[38] found that women in an 8.15am aerobics class achieved a 50%

boost to their feelings of wellbeing compared with 20% for those who worked out at 7.15pm.

There is also evidence that if you exercise before breakfast, in the fasted state, you will burn more fat.

The truth is we are all different and the best time to exercise is the time that best suits you. My optimal time is after the school run and before I settle down into my tunnel of work. I get up and get dressed in my exercise kit so that I'm ready to start exercising as soon as I get home. I've made it part of my routine so that there's less chance of my talking myself out of it.

Michael, on the other hand, splits his exercise. He does his Fast Strength exercises in the morning when he gets out of bed (he finds that if he doesn't do them then he often forgets to do them at all). He gets his HIT in the early evening, by doing Fast Fitness training either on his bike on his way back from work or when he gets home.

What all experts agree is that exercise at any time is better than none at all and that consistency is key to progress. American studies have shown that there are significant benefits to be gained from working out at the same time each day – interestingly, weight lifters who trained at the same time each day consistently gained more power than those who worked out at different times – probably because they were more likely to keep at it.[39]

# Are some people hardwired
## to hate exercise?

We've already discussed research which suggests that the amount of benefit we get from exercise is to some extent hardwired into our genes. The same may well be true of the amount of pleasure we get from exercise.

You might think that if exercise is as good for us as everyone claims we should all be primed to love it. The problem is that from an evolutionary perspective there was never any need to make exercise as enjoyable as sex or food. In the past there was no survival advantage in going for a run or doing press-ups. That would have been a waste of valuable energy at a time when calories were scarce. Our ancestors got all the 'exercise' they needed from simply surviving.

Studies have shown that while some people find exercise enjoyable, for others the opposite is true; they seem to be predisposed to respond more negatively to puffing and panting than others and their mood plummets if they are forced to do it. The result? They throw in the towel early.

The beauty of Fast Exercise is that it is over quickly. So for those who are not blessed with a love of exercise it's a method that may be more sustainable. Certainly the HIT studies show that, though it is demanding, people prefer it to the standard, prolonged slog.

That said, most people need help if they are to stick to a new exercise regime, however short. Fortunately, just as we can train our bodies to become more efficient, so we can coax our minds to become more focused and to respond better to motivational triggers.

## How to keep going

Starting something new is easy. It's keeping going that's hard. It helps, before you start, to be SMART about your reasons for doing an exercise regime. Thoughts like 'I'd quite like to lose some weight' or 'It would be nice to be a bit fitter' are not going to keep you motivated when you are tempted to lie in bed a little bit longer or take the car rather than walking. So make it:

**Specific:** Think about what exactly you are going to do. Specify which days and what time you are going to exercise, and give some serious thought to ensuring that it will be sustainable. If on Tuesdays you tend to work late, for example, don't put a session down for then.

**Measurable:** Blood markers? Waist size? VO2 max? Keep an exercise diary in which you record your baseline statistics re performance, fitness or health, or simply the number of sessions you manage to complete in a week. Michael keeps a really fat photo of himself looking particularly unfit as a reminder.

**Attainable:** Goals need to be realistic and achievable. You are not going to change from an exercise-hating couch potato to a gym bunny overnight. Instead of 'I will lose 10lb', say 'I will take the stairs at work every day this week.'

**Rewarding:** Celebrate your achievements (even just getting started). Treat yourself (though not with a muffin). Share your success with others.

**Time specific:** Commit to doing your chosen regime for at least 3 months. Once you see change you are more likely to keep going.

## Strategies while exercising

We cope with the psychological pressures of exercising in 1 of 2 ways: either we tune into our bodies and focus on what we are doing or we dissociate, think of other things, and generally try to distract ourselves.

Personally, I am what sports psychologists call an 'associator' – I can run for miles without getting bored and without needing to distract myself – to 'dissociate' by using music or other techniques. The good thing about HIT is that most people find that it requires such focus that there's no opportunity to get bored. Self-affirming mantras certainly help. If you need an extra kick to keep going, try shouting to yourself: 'Go for it!', 'Keep going', 'Go, go, GO, GO!!!!', 'Nearly there', 'Not much longer', 'I can get through this'.

Pay attention to the parts of your body which are putting in the most effort, such as your legs when pedalling or running. This will help you keep up the pace and rhythm. As you become tired, it can help to reframe or reinterpret the feeling. 'This burning in my thighs is good – it means I am clearing out my arteries, burning some fat.'

Maintaining your focus also means that you are more likely to hear warning signals coming from your body, telling you that you are pushing it too hard. Some days you just need to be gentle with yourself.

## Eight ways to overcome your inner couch potato

HIT is incredibly time-efficient but even so there will always be reasons not to do it. Here are some of my tips:

1. Write a pledge along the lines of 'I will do a 10-minute session of HIT on the exercise bike, 3 times a week starting tomorrow evening when I get back from work.' Pin it on the wall, schedule it into your diary, put reminders on your phone. Whatever works for you, but the more clearly you have thought it through, the more likely you are to actually do it.

2. Tell those around you what you intend to do and when. Publicly stating a goal makes you more likely to follow through.

3. Exercise with others. If you are planning on going for a jog with added HIT or perhaps you want to do a bit of Fast Walking, find someone to do it with. One of the main reasons people employ trainers is to get them out of the house when they don't feel like going.

4. Join a group or a club. Set up a local group to meet regularly and exercise in the park. But don't be too ambitious as it may become another barrier to getting going. Michael says his mother has talked about joining a walking group for 30 years. She hasn't done it yet.

5. Write a list of potential excuses: can't find shoes,

running clothes in the wash, I'm tired, it's cold, I'll do it tomorrow, the dog has just been sick... Now address each in turn and write down the solutions. If you anticipate potential barriers, it reduces the chance of back-sliding.

6. Create visual cues. Just as you are more likely to eat biscuits if they are in full view, so you are more likely to exercise if the cues are staring you in the face. Put your running shoes by the front door, move the exercise bike into the family room, find somewhere else to hang your washing other than on the cross-trainer.

7. Be aware that you have an inner voice that will tell you 'this is a waste of time'. Remind yourself of your goals. Remind yourself that you will feel better afterwards. Or simply think of something else. Your inner voice is not something you have to pay attention to.

8. Your barriers will be different from mine. But they do need to be considered and also reviewed once you have started the programme. Auditing your experience will make it easier to get in the habit of doing it regularly.

# Food & Fast Exercise

As any committed exerciser or gym member will know, there's an entire industry of energy bars and sports drinks, recovery fluids and protein shakes out there. The good news? You don't need any of them to perform Fast Exercise. Here, instead, are a simple few dos and don'ts:

★ Don't attempt Fast Exercise immediately after eating. This may seem pretty obvious, but the main risk is not cramping, it's vomiting. Michael likes to do his HIT on the way home in the evening, or soon after he gets home. HIT also stops him snacking.

★ Don't load up on carbs before doing Fast Exercise. There is a widespread belief that carbs are needed to fuel exercise. Unless you are exercising heavily for over an hour at a time you have plenty of carbohydrates on board. Eating lots of pasta will simply make you fat.

★ Similarly, you don't need to load up on carbs *after* doing Fast Exercise. You may feel a bit wobbly but the whole point is to deplete your glycogen stores, so the last thing you want to do is immediately replenish them. The average person doing a HIT session 3 times a week does not require special 'refuelling'.

★ As for liquids, doing Fast Exercise is not going to make you sweat so you are unlikely to need to drink during a session. Obviously, drink if you are thirsty. But beware of sports drinks – they are just expensive sugar. If you have been out for a long run and sweated a lot, the best way to rehydrate is with skimmed milk or water.

So is there anything out there that will actually help Fast Exercisers? Well, there are a few foods and drinks with some science behind them, as I outline below (though none of them are things I'm going to be topping myself up with on a regular basis…)

**Beetroot juice:** Beetroot juice is rich in nitrates which increases the levels of nitric oxide in the body. Nitric oxide affects a range of things, including blood flow and cell signalling. Scientists at the University of Exeter found that volunteers who drank 500ml of beetroot juice a day for a week could keep going for longer before getting tired. We may yet see beetroot-loaded athletes at the next Olympics. Beetroot juice is an acquired taste.

**Cherry juice:** Studies at Northumbria University showed that drinking tart cherry juice twice a day for 5 days before a marathon resulted in quicker recovery and less muscle pain after the event. The phytochemicals, especially anthocyanins, found in sour Montmorency cherries in particular have anti-inflammatory and anti-oxidating properties which seem to aid recovery. However, the benefits are clear only in endurance runners. For the rest of us it's just calories.

**Bicarbonate of soda:** Another unlikely drink that might benefit top athletes but which is unlikely to help the rest of us is bicarbonate of soda. In a small study some swimmers who took baking soda an hour before a 200-metre event shaved a second or so off their usual performances. If you are keen then about 20g should do it, in a little water, before exercise and on an empty stomach. Potential soda dopers should be warned that it tastes vile and can cause upset stomachs.

**Ginger:** Ginger root is known to have anti-inflammatory and pain-relieving effects and a randomised controlled study done at the University of Georgia[40] showed that daily ginger consumption reduces muscle pain after exercise. Subjects were asked to take ginger capsules or a placebo for 11 consecutive days and then to perform a series of tough exercises on the eighth day. Ginger supplementation reduced exercise-induced pain by 25%. It's certainly better than taking ibuprofen.

# Kids and HIT

We can learn a lot from children. If you have ever spent time in a primary school playground or at a play park, you will have witnessed the most unadulterated display of HIT-style exercise in action. For children of 10 and under, HIT comes naturally.

I have watched my own 8-year-old son sprint and recover his way around a walk with our Border Collie, perfectly unaware that he is performing the kind of exercise that is taking the scientific world by storm. At that age their bodies are physiologically primed to move fast in short bursts. Young aerobic systems switch on more quickly than those of adults, producing the energy needed for movement, regardless of its intensity. And children's short attention spans mean they are perfectly suited to the stop-start style of Fast Exercise.

But this doesn't mean they should be performing HIT workouts such as those outlined in this book. Structured exercise at a young age should be limited to the occasional football or netball game. Children need to engage in activity freely and uninhibitedly, without pressure and without a stopwatch – indeed, without realising they are doing it at all.

Kids are a good example to us all. Not only are they natural Fast Exercisers, they tend to move about and fidget a lot. And this, as Michael will outline in the next chapter, is key. While HIT is all well and good, it's not enough on its own. The ideal is to combine it with being generally more active.

# MICHAEL'S GUIDE TO
# KEEPING ACTIVE

You might want to read this section of the book while standing up. Or perhaps while strolling around. Remember that the hunter-gatherer approach, which we encountered in Chapter 2, involves much more than simply doing short bursts of intense exercise. It also means increasing the amount of activity that you build into your everyday life. It is the combination of the two that will have a dramatic effect on your health, fitness, weight and welbeing.

All of us have benefited from the technological advances that have occurred in our lifetimes. Our homes are packed full of labour-saving devices. We love our smart phones, email and TVs. But technology also has a lot to answer for. It has made us unbelievably slothful.

Do you know – though why would you – what the average waist-size of a middle-aged woman was in the 1950s? An impressively svelte 28 inches. And now? 34 inches. That 6-inch expansion – 6 inches of unrequired and unloved fat – is partly due to the fact that modern women do not burn anything like as many calories doing housework as their grandmothers did. This is not because women have become more slovenly or, I might add, because men have stepped up to the mark and are doing more around the house – no, men are pretty much as idle around the house as they were a generation ago. The problem is those lovely labour-saving devices.

Sixty years ago a woman could comfortably burn her way through 1,000 calories a day just by doing the chores – washing, mopping and cleaning. These days we let machines take the strain. Very few people would wish to wind back the clock, but somehow we have to find a way to increase the calorie consumption in our lives.

## Ditch the chair

Guess how many hours a day you spend sitting? Less than 8? More than 10? Some experts claim that many of us spend up to 12 hours a day sitting on our well-padded bottoms looking at computers or watching television. If you throw in the 8 hours we spend sleeping, then that adds up to a remarkable 20 hours a day being sedentary. Ouch.

The trouble is that we all kid ourselves about how much we move. To find out just how much, or little, I move in an average day I met up with the incredibly enthusiastic and hyperactive Jim Levine. Jim, who is a professor of medicine at the Mayo Clinic in the US, has had a life-long passion for studying movement. When he was young he would measure the average speed that slugs and snails travelled around in his garden. He is still studying the slothful and sluggardly, but these days he has more sophisticated equipment and his subjects are larger. Much larger.

According to Jim, an obesity specialist, the secret of a long and healthy life lies in improving what he calls your NEAT, your Non Exercise Activity Thermogenesis. As Jim explained, NEAT is about the calories we burn through ordinary everyday living – getting up in the morning, going to bed at night, and all the movements you do while you're sleeping.

To keep the fuels moving through our systems we need to be moving every half an hour or so. And yet, as Jim told me, many of us now regularly spend 12 hours a day in a chair. It is an extraordinary statistic.

'Sedentariness alone appears to be a killer,' he said. 'Bound to the chair, chained to the chair... it's hurting our bodies, it's literally killing millions. Who'd have ever thought that the chair could kill?'

The trouble is that being seated doesn't just burn a bare minimum of calories – sinister things happen when we are inactive for too long. Prolonged sitting has been linked to a sharp reduction in the activity of an important enzyme called lipoprotein lipase which breaks down blood fats and makes them available as a fuel to the muscles. This reduction in enzyme activity leads to raised levels of triglycerides and fats in the blood, increasing the risk of heart disease. Extended sitting has also been shown to cause sharp spikes in blood sugar levels after meals, creating the perfect setting for Type 2 diabetes

Now, I think of myself as quite active, and I found it hard to believe that I was as slothful as Jim suggested. Twelve hours a day sitting down? I challenged him to prove it. At which point he pulled out of his smart leather briefcase a pair of the most extraordinary underpants I have ever seen.

'This,' Jim explained, 'is NEAT underwear, known more colloquially as fidget pants.'

The pants are fitted with multiple sensors and accelerometers designed to detect – and to store on a microprocessor – every movement made by the wearer. 'So if you wear these for a day,' Jim continued, 'we can see everything you were doing 20 times a second, night and day.'

Two weeks later, we met up again to get the results, standing up of course. Jim's reaction was not encouraging. 'Oh dear, oh dear, oh dear!' he said. Apparently my fidget pants had revealed that in an average day there was not a lot of fidgeting going on at all. There was move, stop, move, stop, but most of it was stop. In fact, Jim's pants suggested I spent at least 11 hours a day sitting down, sometimes for several hours at a time. During long meetings I became positively comatose.

This was sobering. I was aware that I spent quite a lot of time sitting and thinking, but certainly not that much. So I decided to see what would happen if I made a deliberate attempt to keep on my feet more.

I put the magic pants back on and for the next 24 hours I made a concerted effort to keep on the move, without actually exercising. I found it impossible to avoid my desk completely, but I did avoid the lift and took every opportunity to get up and just stroll around a bit, brainstorming with colleagues while on the move.

When I returned a while later, pants in hand, Jim was extremely encouraging. 'Congratulations,' he said, 'you doubled your amount of NEAT. I mean, we're talking 500 extra calories burnt in one day through some simple changes. And how much sweat did you drip doing this? I'm betting none...'

Keeping on the move isn't just a good way of burning calories. It also has a big impact on your health. In a recent study from Australia[41] researchers gathered 70 healthy adults and asked them to do a series of experiments which involved an awful lot of sitting.

In the first part of the experiment they were asked to sit for 9 hours straight. Every few hours they were asked to knock back a meal replacement drink. Soon after having their delicious drink they had their blood glucose levels and insulin levels measured.

Then they did it all over again, exactly the same, except

this time they were asked to walk around at a brisk pace for half an hour before they did a 9-hour sitting stint.

They were then asked to do it one final time, except on this occasion they had to get up and walk around for exactly 1 minute and 40 seconds every 30 minutes.

On analysing the data, the researchers discovered that when the volunteers got up and walked every half-hour their bodies were much better at coping with the meal replacement drinks. There wasn't the same surge in either glucose or insulin that they saw when the volunteers just sat. In fact, their blood glucose levels went down by 39%, while their insulin levels also fell by an impressive 26%.

What this and other studies clearly show is that we need to move more. Short bursts of activity can be as effective as much longer periods of continuous activity at improving sugar and fat levels.

So if you do spend a lot of your work life sitting down, find an excuse to get up and move – every 30 minutes.

## Where are the stairs?

There are many ways in which modern society conspires to keep us burning as few calories as possible, the most obvious example being the car. But one of my particular beefs is stairs. Why are buildings designed so that the stairs are so incredibly hard to find and use? I try to take the stairs as often as I can, but all too frequently they are hidden somewhere inaccessible. And they're usually uninviting too.

Escalators and walkways are just as bad. As soon as people step on an escalator they freeze, blocking the way for everyone else. The really depressing thing is that despite what we know about the benefits of keeping moving, modern architectural design seems to be taking us in the opposite direction.

When sports scientists at Loughborough University looked at the availability of stairs in newly built shopping centres, airports and other public places, they found there were pitifully few. Architects design new buildings with escalators and lifts to comply with access requirements – in which the stairs are not there to be used, except in a fire evacuation.

Yet as Professor Gregory Heath, from the School of Public Health at the University of Tennessee, has repeatedly pointed out, one of the best ways to make people more active is to provide motivational signs directing them to use the stairs instead of the lifts. It only works, of course, if they can find them.

Our advice? Find the stairs, and use them whenever you can. They are not just for HIT. You can also use them to move from floor to floor.

# 10,000 steps

The easiest way to get more active is to walk. As I mentioned earlier, a typical hunter-gatherer walks 6-10km a day. That comes to roughly 10,000 steps, the currently recommended level of activity that we should all be aiming at. Many of us don't get close.

In *The Step Diet*,[42] the authors quote a Harris poll in which 1,000 Americans were asked to wear step counters (pedometers) for two days. They found that people who were overweight walked nearly 2,000 fewer steps a day than those who were slimmer and that half of all women over 50 didn't reach even half the recommended levels (men did slightly better).

Walking will only burn modest numbers of calories, but if you do enough and on a regular basis it all adds up. Walking also has other, more subtle benefits – not the least of which is that, unlike jogging, it does not seem to lead to compensatory eating.

To discover just how much difference walking can make I took part in an unusual experiment organised by Dr Jason Gill of Glasgow University.

We met on a cold winter's morning in a Scottish café where Jason suggested I eat a large breakfast. Bacon, eggs, sausages and bread, all fried in butter and oil.

'The amount of fat in that breakfast,' he told me, 'is similar to the amount of fat people eat during the course of a day. The fat's going to go into your gut, and then into your bloodstream, where it's going to cause a number of changes to your metabolism, and all these things are going to increase the risk of fatty deposits forming on the walls of your blood vessels.'

I paused, fork halfway to my mouth, to digest this thought. 'If you think that sounds bad,' he added helpfully, 'wait till you see it.'

Four hours after my breakfast Jason took a sample of my blood, which he then spun in a high-speed centrifuge to separate the various elements. 'That's the fat from the food that you've eaten, right there,' he said, pointing to a creamy, milky fluid sitting at the top of the test tube. 'That's the stuff that's been circulating round your body for the last couple of hours. If we compare this with a blood sample taken before you ate breakfast you can see that eating all that fried food has doubled the amount of fat in your bloodstream.'

Slightly shaken, I headed off for a walk. Jason assured me that walking even a few miles would make a measurable difference.

The next morning I went back to the same café to complete part two of the experiment. I ate exactly the same meal. Four hours after eating, Jason again took a sample of my blood and after much spinning and separating presented me with the results.

'You can see,' he said, 'that there's substantially less fat in the sample today than there was yesterday. Today you've got about a third less fat going round your bloodstream, a third less fat interacting with the walls of your blood vessels.'

The walking I had done the previous afternoon had switched on genes that make an enzyme called lipoprotein lipase, and it was this enzyme that produced the striking 33% fall in the amount of circulating fat. I was impressed and immediately went out and bought a pedometer.

These days whenever I'm tempted to drive a short distance that I could easily walk I remember Jason's test tubes.

## High intensity interval walking – Fast Walking

Walking is good, but Fast Walking is better. Like other forms of Fast activity, Fast Walking involves alternating walking fast with walking slow.

In a recent study published in *Diabetes Care*,[43] 24 volunteers with Type 2 diabetes were asked to walk for an hour a day, 5 days a week. Twelve of them were asked to walk at a constant speed, the other 12 alternated 3 minutes of brisk walking with 3 minutes of gentle walking. The volunteers all wore accelerometers and heart-rate monitors to ensure that both groups were doing the same amount of work, burning the same number of calories.

At the end of the 4-month trial they found that the volunteers who had done Fast Walking had improved their VO2 max by 16%, lost fat and improved their blood glucose control. The changes were far greater than in those who had walked at a constant speed.

In another study from Japan[44] involving 248 men and women in which researchers compared 3 minutes' fast-slow walking with continuous speed walking, they again saw much greater improvements in the Fast Walking group. In this study the volunteers did 5 bursts of Fast Walking a day, 4 days a week.

For suggestions on how to do a Fast Walking workout see page 121.

## 12 easy ways to introduce more activity into our lives

The following suggestions come mainly from the Mayo clinic, where Professor Jim Levine is based.

1. Stand while talking on the phone. You'll burn calories and sound more assertive.
2. If you work at a desk for long periods you might consider buying a standing desk. This is a desk at which, as the name implies, you stand. Winston Churchill apparently wrote some of his famous speeches while working at one.

3. If you have to sit, try using a chair with no back, or even one of those giant sit-on balls. This strenghens core muscles and prevents slumping (and therefore backache).
4. Go and see a colleague instead of sending an email.
5. Walk laps with the other members of a meeting rather than gather in a conference room.
6. Drink lots of water. This not only keeps you hydrated but it also increases the need for bathroom breaks, which means in turn more short, brisk walks.
7. Rather than taking a break with a coffee or a snack, take a stroll or go up and down the stairs.
8. If you normally take a bus or train to work, get off at an earlier stop than usual and walk the rest of the way.
9. If you drive to work, park at the far end of the car park.
10. Keep resistance bands – stretchy cords or tubes that offer resistance when you pull on them – or small hand weights near your desk. Do arm curls between meetings or tasks.
11. Organise a lunchtime walking group. You might be surrounded by people who are just dying to lace up their trainers. Enjoy the camaraderie, and offer encouragement to one another when you feel like back-sliding.
12. If you're stuck in an airport, don't sit down. Grab your bags and go look around the shops.

## In summary...

We cannot stress enough that Fast Exercise will be fully effective only if you lead an otherwise active life. One of the dispiriting things that happen as we get older is that we tend, almost imperceptibly, to put on weight. The pounds creep up on us – generally at a rate of 2-3lb (1-1.5kg) a year  barely noticeable at first, but eventually forcing us up a whole size in clothes. Much of this gain is down to general inactivity.

On average, thin people stand for around 2 hours longer every day than those who carry more weight. Simply by standing more, pacing around a bit more, taking the stairs and walking when you can, you should burn through at least an extra 350 calories a day. Over a year this adds up to the calorie equivalent of running about 1,000 miles.

# BEFORE YOU GO...

As we've seen, the science of exercise is moving fast. HIT – ultra-short bursts of intense activity – has been shown to be an extremely time-efficient way to improve fitness and health, particularly when combined (as in the hunter-gatherer approach) with increased levels of general activity; and its use is gradually extending, from athletes and the young and healthy to those who are older and less fit.

As with all forms of exercise it's important not to overdo or rush into HIT; but I find it encouraging (and surprising) that so far its safety and effectiveness have stood up to being tested in people who are most at risk, those with a history of heart disease and stroke.

The joy of Fast Exercise, of course, is that the exertion is short-lived: it is the perfect workout for the time-starved generation. It can fit unobtrusively into your day – so much so that, if you stick with it, it soon becomes habitual.

There are few miracles in this world, and this book is not offering you a magic wand. What we recommend is rather a shift in your perception, so that you come to see exercise not as an unwelcome chore to be got over and done with – yet another thing on your To Do list, to be slotted in at the end of a hard week – but instead as a small, but key part of your daily life, an activity almost as instinctual as getting up in the morning and brushing your teeth. In this way, Fast Exercise should become sustainable and, dare I say it, even enjoyable.

And this is the case whether you are an aerobic high responder who already enjoys doing lots of exercise, like Peta, or a low responder who does not, like me.

For high responders, HIT offers a rapid, high-impact regime that can be added to existing workouts to maximise their effectiveness. For the sloths among us, HIT is a joy because it liberates us from the hell of slogging round the running track or going to the gym (which, let's be honest, we are never going to do), while still delivering many of the other wonders of exercise, including increased fat burning. Though be aware that without watching your calories no exercise regime will ever lead to long-term weight loss.

So far studies on HIT have largely been confined to athletes, hospitals and the laboratory. Plans are underway to study its effectiveness in real-life settings, particularly in the workplace. I await the results of those studies with interest.

Another area of research that this book has tried to highlight is the danger of the chair. The chair is not simply a useful bit of furniture, it is a killer. Instead of spending hours at a time hunched over our computers or televisions, allowing the sugar and fat from our last meal to clog up our arteries, we need to recognise the importance of intermittent movement, to find reasons to get up from our chairs and go for a short stroll or even just have a brief stretch at least once every half-hour.

The fact that we are becoming increasingly sedentary, with all the problems that this leads to (increased risk of diabetes, heart disease, dementia, to name but a few), is surely evidence that public exhortations and health messages are not enough. We need help to overcome our inner sloth. And some of this needs has to come from above. There are examples, though not nearly enough, of cities where politicians, architects, planners and employers have come together to make changes to the physical environment – changes that encourage us to burn calories rather than simply add them to our burgeoning bellies. We need more city centres where it is safe to cycle and where cars are banned or severely limited; buildings with stairs that are visible, attractive and inviting to use; escalators that invite us to walk rather than stay rooted to the spot.

We were born to move. Some of us more reluctantly than others. So let's find ways to do it more. Fast.

# WAYS TO MEASURE
# THE IMPACT OF EXERCISE

You can do the following calculations yourself or visit our website, **fast-exercises.com**, where you can obtain more information, get the calculations done automatically and join a forum to discuss all things exercise-related.

## The importance of heart rate

Your resting heart rate is itself a powerful predictor of future health. According to a study of 11,000 people published in *The Lancet* (September 2008), those with heart rates above 70 beats per minute are at greater risk of heart attack and hospital admission. With regular exercise you should see your resting heart rate fall.

Top athletes can have a resting pulse as low as 40 beats per minute. Mine is around 64 beats per minute.

Your resting heart rate is easy to find. Turn your hand so your palm is facing you. Use your index and middle finger from your other hand to measure it at the wrist, just below the thumb. Measure it when you are sitting down and relaxed, preferably first thing in the morning.

# Heart rate max (HR max)

Some of the exercises in this book talk about pushing yourself to 80% or 90% of your maximum heart rate. So how do you measure that? The most direct way is to run or cycle as fast as you can against resistance for about 3 minutes, rest for a couple of minutes, then try pushing yourself as hard as possible for another couple of minutes. Your heart rate will probably peak at some point during the second burst. This should not be attempted if you have any doubts about your fitness.

When I did it, the highest I could get my heart rate to was 164, so my HR max is 164.

If you prefer something less stressful, the safest way to get an estimate of your HR max is by using one of the formulae for calculating it, of which the best known is 220 minus your age for men and 226 minus your age for women. It is simple, but out of date, and a more reliable version for both sexes is HR max = $205.8 - (0.685 \times age)$.

On this basis my HR max is 167, which is close to what I found in practice.

Knowing your HR max will help you calculate how hard to push yourself when you are doing some of the HIT exercises in the book, though you will probably also need a heart-rate monitor as stopping to measure your heart rate while you are exercising is tricky.

HR max will also help you calculate your VO2 max.

# VO2 max

VO2 max is a measure of aerobic fitness, one of the most important predictors of future health. The most reliable way to find your VO2 max is to have it done in a lab or a gym that has suitable facilities. But if you don't have access to a lab there are other ways to estimate your aerobic fitness.

The simplest is the Uth–Sørensen–Overgaard–Pedersen estimation:

$$\text{VO2 max} = 15.3 \times \text{HR max/HR rest}$$

Since my HR max is 164 and my resting heart rate is 64, according to this formula my VO2 max $= 15.3 \times 164/64 = 39.2$ mL/(kg·min).

This is reasonably close to the result I got when my VO2 max was tested in the lab, which was 37 mL/(kg·min). (Just to put that in perspective: Peta's VO2 max is a whopping 53 mL/(kg·min), which is very high for a woman, let alone one of her age. Actually, by my standards, it's high for a man too.)

Once you have estimated your VO2 max use the charts overleaf, to see how well you are doing. For my age I am rated 'good'.

Unless you are an aerobic non-responder you should see improvements in your VO2 max after 6 weeks of following a Fast Exercise regime.

## WOMEN

| Age (years) | Very poor | Poor | Fair | Average | Good | Very good | Excellent |
|---|---|---|---|---|---|---|---|
| 20-24 | < 27 | 27-31 | 32-36 | 37-41 | 42-46 | 47-51 | > 51 |
| 25-29 | < 26 | 26-30 | 31-35 | 36-40 | 41-44 | 45-49 | > 49 |
| 30-34 | < 25 | 25-29 | 30-33 | 34-37 | 38-42 | 43-46 | > 46 |
| 35-39 | < 24 | 24-27 | 28-31 | 32-35 | 36-40 | 41-44 | > 44 |
| 40-44 | < 22 | 22-25 | 26-29 | 30-33 | 34-37 | 38-41 | > 41 |
| 45-49 | < 21 | 21-23 | 24-27 | 28-31 | 32-35 | 36-38 | > 38 |
| 50-54 | < 19 | 19-22 | 23-25 | 26-29 | 30-32 | 33-36 | > 36 |
| 55-59 | < 18 | 18-20 | 21-23 | 24-27 | 28-30 | 31-33 | > 33 |
| 60-65 | < 16 | 16-18 | 19-21 | 22-24 | 25-27 | 28-30 | > 30 |

## MEN

| Age (years) | Very poor | Poor | Fair | Average | Good | Very good | Excellent |
|---|---|---|---|---|---|---|---|
| 20-24 | < 32 | 32-37 | 38-43 | 44-50 | 51-56 | 57-62 | > 62 |
| 25-29 | < 31 | 31-35 | 36-42 | 43-48 | 49-53 | 54-59 | > 59 |
| 30-34 | < 29 | 29-34 | 35-40 | 41-45 | 46-51 | 52-56 | > 56 |
| 35-39 | < 28 | 28-32 | 33-38 | 39-43 | 44-48 | 49-54 | > 54 |
| 40-44 | < 26 | 26-31 | 32-35 | 36-41 | 42-46 | 47-51 | > 51 |
| 45-49 | < 25 | 25-29 | 30-34 | 35-39 | 40-43 | 44-48 | > 48 |
| 50-54 | < 24 | 24-27 | 28-32 | 33-36 | 37-41 | 42-46 | > 46 |
| 55-59 | < 22 | 22-26 | 27-30 | 31-34 | 35-39 | 40-43 | > 43 |
| 60-65 | < 21 | 21-24 | 25-28 | 29-32 | 33-36 | 37-40 | > 40 |

# The Rockport one mile walk test

This is a better way of estimating VO2 max. You walk a mile as briskly as you can, then measure your heart rate at the end.

### The formula:
VO2 max = 132.853 – (0.0769 × Weight) – (0.3877 × Age) + (6.315 × Gender) – (3.2649 × Time) – (0.1565 × Heart rate)

1. You enter your weight in pounds (lb).
2. Gender male = 1 and female = 0.
3. You measure the time you take to walk the mile in minutes and seconds.

I'm 164lb, 56 years old, male. I did the walk in 14 minutes and 30 seconds (14.5 mins) and my heart rate was 120 beats per min at the end:

VO2 max = 133 – (0.0769 ×164) – (0.3877 × 56) + (6.315 × 1) – (3.2649 × 14.5) – (0.1565 × 120) = 132 – 12.7 – 21.7 + 6.3 – 47.3 – 18.8 = 37.8

# Alternative ways of
## assessing aerobic fitness

## *The Cooper Run*

Another long-standing test was devised for the US Air Force by physiologist Kenneth Cooper and first published in the *Journal of the American Medical Association* back in 1968. It is still widely used by athletes and football teams. In its original form the test requires you to run as far as you can in 12 minutes on a 400-metre athletics track (so that distance can be measured accurately to the nearest 10 metres). Your aerobic fitness can then be estimated from the following table:

| COOPER TEST (20-50+) | | Very Good | Good | Average | Bad | Very Bad |
|---|---|---|---|---|---|---|
| 20-29 | M | 2800+m | 2400-2800m | 2200-2399m | 1600-2199m | 1600-m |
| | F | 2700+m | 2200-2700m | 1800-2199m | 1500-1799m | 1500-m |
| 30-39 | M | 2700+m | 2300-2700m | 1900-2299m | 1500-1899m | 1500-m |
| | F | 2500+m | 2000-2500m | 1700-1999m | 1400-1699m | 1400-m |
| 40-49 | M | 2500+m | 2100-2500m | 1700-2099m | 1400 -1699m | 1400-m |
| | F | 2300+m | 1900-2300m | 1500-1899m | 1200-1499m | 1200-m |
| 50+ | M | 2400+m | 2000-2400m | 1600-1999m | 1300-1599m | 1300-m |
| | F | 2200+m | 1700-2200m | 1400-1699m | 1100-1399m | 1100-m |

| COOPER TEST (Experienced athletes) | | | | | | |
|---|---|---|---|---|---|---|
| | M | 3700+m | 3400-3700m | 3100-3399m | 2800-3099m | 2800-m |
| | F | 3000+m | 2700-3000m | 2400-2699m | 2100-2399m | 2100-m |

## Oral glucose tolerance test

One of the most important things that regular exercise does is help your body cope with high levels of blood glucose after a meal.

Persistently elevated blood sugar, even if it isn't in the diabetic range, is a bad sign. Unless it is removed, excess glucose binds to body proteins (a process called glycation), damaging arteries and nerves. This, in turn, can lead to blindness, impotence, dementia and heart disease.

The oral glucose tolerance test is an important measure of your metabolic fitness, how well and how quickly your body deals with glucose. It is a test that is best done by your doctor but it can also be done at home – though this should not be attempted at home if you are a Type 1 or Type 2 diabetic, if you suffer from needle phobia, or have any reason to believe you will respond badly to a significant sugar hit.

The test consists of consuming 75gm of fast-acting carbohydate, either as a drink or as food, on an empty stomach, then measuring the effects that has on your blood glucose levels.

If you are doing it at home, then first you have to buy a simple blood glucose monitoring kit from your chemist or online.

- **You need to fast overnight for a minimum of 10 hours (only water permitted).**

• You then dissolve 75g of glucose in 300ml of water. You can buy glucose from a chemist or online. Ordinary table sugar, sucrose, is made up of glucose and fructose, so it is not the same. It needs to be drunk within a couple of minutes.

• Alternatively you can drink 380ml of Lucozade Original.

• If you prefer, 8oz (240gm) of boiled potato will deliver roughly the same level of carbohydrate. Nothing else to be eaten with it, though.

• The main thing is be consistent if you decide to repeat the test months later.

Once you've drunk glucose or eaten the potato, record the time. At the end of 1 hour, and then again at 2 hours, prick your finger and measure your blood glucose levels, recording the results.

## How to interpret the results

Too high? By the end of 2 hours your glucose levels should have fallen below 7.4mmol/L (120mg/dl). If that hasn't happened then you may be diabetic or have impaired glucose tolerance. See your doctor, who will probably repeat the tests in a more controlled setting.

Too low? If your blood sugar goes high after 1 hour but then drops below 3.9mmol/L (70mg/dl) at 2 hours you may have 'reactive hypoglycemia'. After drinking the glucose or eating the carbs your blood sugar went up, so your pancreas pumped out insulin to bring it down. But it was too much so you ended up with low blood sugar. The symptoms are wide ranging but may include fatigue and dizziness. Again, see your doctor.

If your blood glucose is elevated, i.e. above 6.1mmol/L (110 mg/dL), then do keep an eye on it. Six weeks of Fast Exercise should improve your body's ability to cope with glucose. Let us know, via the website, how you get on.

# Muscular Fitness

Doing regular Fast Strength exercises should, depending on your genes, make you stronger. One way of assessing this is by the number of press-ups you can do in 1 minute. If you are unfit (or a woman) you may want to start with a modified press-up, kneeling down and then pushing yourself up.

The following chart is based on research done – like the aerobic fitness test, above – at the Cooper Institute for Aerobics Research in Dallas, Texas, where they have collected data on over 100,000 people. As I mentioned, Kenneth Cooper was an Air Force doctor who carried out some of the first extensive research on aerobic exercise and wrote a bestseller, *Aerobics*, in 1968. Among other groups, the Cooper Institute work with the military and the police. Apparently American policemen tend to be overweight, aerobically unfit, but stronger than the average person.

MEN: Full body press-ups

| Age | 20-29 | 30-39 | 40-49 | 50-59 | 60+ |
|---|---|---|---|---|---|
| Superior | 62 | 52 | 40 | 39 | 28 |
| Excellent | 47 | 39 | 30 | 35 | 23 |
| Good | 37 | 30 | 24 | 19 | 18 |
| Fair | 29 | 24 | 18 | 13 | 10 |
| Poor | 22 | 17 | 11 | 9 | 6 |
| Very poor | 13 | 9 | 5 | 3 | 2 |

## WOMEN: Modified press-ups

| Age | 20-29 | 30-39 | 40-49 | 50-59 | 60+ |
|---|---|---|---|---|---|
| Superior | 45 | 39 | 33 | 28 | 20 |
| Excellent | 36 | 31 | 24 | 21 | 15 |
| Good | 30 | 24 | 18 | 17 | 12 |
| Fair | 23 | 19 | 13 | 12 | 5 |
| Poor | 7 | 11 | 6 | 6 | 2 |
| Very poor | 9 | 4 | 1 | 0 | 0 |

## WOMEN: Full press-ups

| Age | 20-29 | 30-39 | 40-49 |
|---|---|---|---|
| Superior | 42 | 39 | 20 |
| Excellent | 28 | 23 | 15 |
| Good | 21 | 15 | 13 |
| Fair | 15 | 11 | 9 |
| Poor | 10 | 8 | 6 |
| Very poor | 3 | 1 | 0 |

I started out in the 'good' range, able to do 20 press-ups in a minute. After a couple of months doing high intensity circuit training, I am now able to do 40 in a minute, which I'm pleased to say pushes me into 'superior'.

Peta, being a runner, has not focused on strength and she is not keen on press-ups. She tells me she can manage about 20 modified press-ups in a minute. 'Good'.

# Get on the scales

An obvious thing you will want to do before embarking on this adventure is to weigh yourself. Initially, it is best to do this at the same time every day. First thing in the morning is, as I'm sure you know, when you will be at your lightest.

Ideally, you should get a weighing machine that measures body-fat percentage as well as weight, since what you really want to see is your body-fat levels fall and muscle rise. The cheaper machines are not fantastically reliable; they tend to underestimate the true figure, giving you a false sense of security. What they are quite good at doing, however, is measuring change. In other words, they might tell you when you start that you are 30% body fat when the true figure is closer to 33%. But they should be able to tell you when that number begins to fall.

## Body fat

Body fat is measured as a percentage of total weight. The machines you can buy do this by a system called impedence. They generate a small electric current that runs through your body and measure the resistance to it. The estimation is based on the fact that muscle and other tissues are better conductors of electricity than fat.

The only way to get a truly accurate figure is with a machine called a DXA (formerly DEXA) scanner. It stands for 'Dual

Energy X-ray Absorptiometry'. It is expensive and for most people unnecessary. Your body mass index (BMA) will tell you if you are overweight. Women tend to have more body fat than men. A man with body fat of more than 25% would be considered overweight. For a woman it would be 30%.

## Calculate your BMI

To calculate your BMI, go to a website, such as: http://www.nhs.uk/Tools/Pages/Healthyweightcalculator.aspx. This will not only do the calculation, but also tell you what it means. One criticism of BMI is that someone who has a lot of muscle could get a high BMI score. This is not an issue for most of us. Sadly.

## Measure your stomach

BMI is useful but it may not be the best predictor of future health. In a study of over 45,000 women followed for 16 years, it was the waist-to-height ratio that proved a superior predictor of who would develop heart disease.

The reason the waist matters so much is because the worst sort of fat is visceral fat, which collects inside the abdomen. Most people think that fat is fat and all fat is equal. Recently it has become clear that this is not true. Subcutaneous fat, the sort of fat you get on your arms, legs and buttocks, is unsightly but has relatively little impact on health. The visceral fat coats and infiltrates your internal organs like your liver and your pancreas. It causes inflammation and puts you at much higher risk of diabetes.

You would imagine that if you had lots of visceral fat you would have to look fat, but this is not the case. I only discovered that I was a TOFI (Thin on the Outside, Fat Inside) when I went for an MRI scan as part of a documentary. I didn't look overweight but the scan revealed that in fact I had many litres of internal fat. Around 25% of people who have a normal BMI will have worrying levels of visceral fat, without knowing it. Although it is not ideal, if you can't afford an MRI or a DXA scan, the simplest and cheapest test is a tape measure.

Male or female, your waist should be less than half your height. Most people underestimate their waist size by about 2 inches because they rely on trouser size. Instead, measure your waist by putting the tape measure around your belly button. Be honest. A definition of optimism is someone who steps on the scales while holding their breath. You are fooling no one.

# Calories burnt doing different activities

This chart is here more for general interest than anything else. I find that when I am tempted to eat a calorie-laden muffin (and I am, regularly), then I just think about how much activity I will have to do to burn off those calories. These figures are gross. To get net calories burnt you have to subtract your basal metabolic rate (BMR), the calories that you would have burnt sitting down doing nothing. Your BMR depends on your age, weight, sex and height. Mine is around 67 calories per hour.

| Activity, Exercise or Sport (1 hour) | 130lb | 155lb | 180lb | 205lb |
|---|---|---|---|---|
| Walking the dog | 177 | 211 | 245 | 279 |
| Squash | 708 | 844 | 981 | 1117 |
| Ballroom dancing, slow | 177 | 211 | 245 | 279 |
| Ballroom dancing, fast | 325 | 387 | 449 | 512 |
| Running upstairs | 885 | 1056 | 1226 | 1396 |
| Archery | 207 | 246 | 286 | 326 |
| Badminton | 266 | 317 | 368 | 419 |
| Basketball | 354 | 422 | 490 | 558 |
| Billiards | 148 | 176 | 204 | 233 |
| Bowling | 177 | 211 | 245 | 279 |
| Cricket (batting, bowling) | 295 | 352 | 409 | 465 |
| Croquet | 148 | 176 | 204 | 233 |

| Activity, Exercise or Sport (1 hour) | 130lb | 155lb | 180lb | 205lb |
|---|---|---|---|---|
| Darts | 148 | 176 | 204 | 233 |
| Fencing | 354 | 422 | 490 | 558 |
| Frisbee playing | 177 | 211 | 245 | 279 |
| Golf, general | 266 | 317 | 368 | 419 |
| Riding a horse | 236 | 281 | 327 | 372 |
| Horse grooming, vigorous | 354 | 422 | 490 | 558 |
| Martial arts, judo, karate, kick-boxing | 590 | 704 | 817 | 931 |
| Juggling | 236 | 281 | 327 | 372 |
| Rock climbing | 649 | 774 | 899 | 1024 |
| Skipping | 590 | 704 | 817 | 931 |
| Skateboarding | 295 | 352 | 409 | 465 |
| Roller skating | 413 | 493 | 572 | 651 |
| Roller blading | 708 | 844 | 981 | 1117 |
| Sky diving | 177 | 211 | 245 | 279 |
| Football, competitive | 590 | 704 | 817 | 931 |
| Football, non-competitive | 413 | 493 | 572 | 651 |
| Table tennis, ping pong | 236 | 281 | 327 | 372 |
| Tai chi | 236 | 281 | 327 | 372 |

| Activity, Exercise or Sport (1 hour) | 130lb | 155lb | 180lb | 205lb |
|---|---|---|---|---|
| Tennis, doubles | 354 | 422 | 490 | 558 |
| Tennis, singles | 472 | 563 | 654 | 745 |
| Trampoline | 207 | 246 | 286 | 326 |
| Volleyball, beach | 472 | 563 | 654 | 745 |
| Backpacking, Hiking | 413 | 493 | 572 | 651 |
| Carrying a child, level ground | 207 | 246 | 286 | 326 |
| Carrying a child, upstairs | 295 | 352 | 409 | 465 |
| Carrying 16 to 24lb, upstairs | 354 | 422 | 490 | 558 |
| Carrying 25 to 49lb, upstairs | 472 | 563 | 654 | 745 |
| Standing, chatting | 165 | 197 | 229 | 261 |
| Walking/running, playing with children, moderate | 236 | 281 | 327 | 372 |
| Loading, unloading car | 177 | 211 | 245 | 279 |
| Climbing hills, carrying up to 9lb | 413 | 493 | 572 | 651 |
| Climbing hills, carrying 10 to 20lb | 443 | 528 | 613 | 698 |
| Climbing hills, carrying 21 to 42lb | 472 | 563 | 654 | 745 |
| Climbing hills, carrying over 42lb | 531 | 633 | 735 | 838 |
| Walking downstairs | 177 | 211 | 245 | 279 |
| Birdwatching | 148 | 176 | 204 | 233 |

| Activity, Exercise or Sport (1 hour) | 130lb | 155lb | 180lb | 205lb |
|---|---|---|---|---|
| Marching, rapidly, military | 384 | 457 | 531 | 605 |
| Children's games like hopscotch, | 295 | 352 | 409 | 465 |
| Pushing stroller or walking with children | 148 | 176 | 204 | 233 |
| Pushing a wheelchair | 236 | 281 | 327 | 372 |
| Walking using crutches | 295 | 352 | 409 | 465 |
| Walking 2.0 mph, slow | 148 | 176 | 204 | 233 |
| Walking 3.0 mph, moderate | 195 | 232 | 270 | 307 |
| Walking 3.5 mph, uphill | 354 | 422 | 490 | 558 |
| Walking 4.0 mph, brisk | 295 | 352 | 409 | 465 |
| Walking 5.0 mph | 472 | 563 | 654 | 745 |
| Boating, power-, speed-boat | 148 | 176 | 204 | 233 |
| Crew, sculling, rowing, competition | 708 | 844 | 981 | 1117 |
| Kayaking | 295 | 352 | 409 | 465 |
| Skiing, water-skiing | 354 | 422 | 490 | 558 |
| Snorkelling | 295 | 352 | 409 | 465 |
| Surfing | 177 | 211 | 245 | 279 |
| Whitewater rafting, kayaking, canoeing | 295 | 352 | 409 | 465 |

| Activity, Exercise or Sport (1 hour) | 130lb | 155lb | 180lb | 205lb |
|---|---|---|---|---|
| Treading water, vigorous | 590 | 704 | 817 | 931 |
| Treading water, moderate | 236 | 281 | 327 | 372 |
| Water aerobics | 236 | 281 | 327 | 372 |
| Water polo | 590 | 704 | 817 | 931 |
| Water volleyball | 177 | 211 | 245 | 279 |
| Diving, springboard or platform | 177 | 211 | 245 | 279 |
| Ice skating, average speed | 413 | 493 | 572 | 651 |
| Sledding, tobagganing | 413 | 493 | 572 | 651 |
| Snowmobiling | 207 | 246 | 286 | 326 |
| General housework | 207 | 246 | 286 | 326 |
| Cleaning gutters | 295 | 352 | 409 | 465 |
| Painting | 266 | 317 | 368 | 419 |
| Sitting, playing with animals | 148 | 176 | 204 | 233 |
| Walking /running, playing with animals | 236 | 281 | 327 | 372 |
| Mowing lawn, walking, power mower | 325 | 387 | 449 | 512 |
| Mowing lawn, riding mower | 148 | 176 | 204 | 233 |
| Shoveling snow by hand | 354 | 422 | 490 | 558 |

| Activity, Exercise or Sport (1 hour) | 130lb | 155lb | 180lb | 205lb |
|---|---|---|---|---|
| Raking lawn | 254 | 303 | 351 | 400 |
| Gardening, general | 236 | 281 | 327 | 372 |
| Watering lawn or garden | 89 | 106 | 123 | 140 |
| Carpentry, general | 207 | 246 | 286 | 326 |
| Carrying heavy loads | 472 | 563 | 654 | 745 |
| Taking out the rubbish | 177 | 211 | 245 | 279 |
| Teaching physical education, exercise class | 236 | 281 | 327 | 372 |
| Teaching & participating in exercise class | 384 | 457 | 531 | 605 |

# ENDNOTES

1.        Non-vigorous physical activity and all-cause mortality: systematic review and meta-analysis of cohort studies. Int J Epidemiol. 2011 Feb;40(1):121-38. doi: 10.1093/ije/dyq104. Epub 2010 Jul 14. Woodcock J, Franco OH, Orsini N, Roberts I.

2.        Using speed of ageing and "microlives" to communicate the effects of lifetime habits and environment BMJ2012;345doi: http://dx.doi.org/10.1136/bmj.e8223 (Published 17 December 2012).

3.        Aerobic Exercise Training Increases Brain Volume in Aging Humans, Colcombe SJ, Erickson KI, Scalf PE, Kim JS, Prakash R, McAuley E, Elavsky S, Marquez DX, Hu L, Kramer AF. J Gerontol A Biol Sci Med Sci. 2006 Nov; 61(11):1166-70.

4.        The Association Between Midlife Cardiorespiratory Fitness Levels and Later-Life Dementia: A Cohort Study. Ann Intern Med 2013 Feb 5; 158:162.

5.        Musculoskeletal dysfunction in physical education teachers. Occup Environ Med 2000;57:673-677. Hélène Sandmark.

6.        Run for Your Life... at a comfortable speed and not too far. "Heart" 2013;99:516-519 doi:10.1136/heartjnl-2012-302886.

7.        Longevity in Male and Female Joggers; American J. Epidemiology. Feb 2013 Peter Schnohr et al.

8.        High serum glucose levels are associated with a higher perceived age Diana van Heemst. AGE February 2013, Volume 35, Issue 1, pp 189-195.

9.        The effect of high-intensity intermittent exercise on body composition of overweight young males. J Obes. 2012;2012:480467. doi: 10.1155/2012/480467. Epub 2012 Jun 6. Heydari M, Freund J, Boutcher SH.

10.        Effect of exercise on 24-month weight loss maintenance

in overweight women. Archives of Internal Medicine, 2008 Jul 28;168(14):1550-9; discussion 1559-60. doi: 10.1001/archinte.168.14.1550. Jakicic JM, Marcus BH, Lang W, Janney C.

11.      Adapted from "Energy Expenditure of Walking and Running," Medicine & Science in Sport & Exercise, Cameron et al, Dec. 2004.

12.      The effects of high-intensity intermittent exercise training on fat loss and fasting insulin levels of young women. Int J Obes (Lond). 2008 Apr;32(4):684-91. doi: 10.1038/sj.ijo.0803781. Epub 2008 Jan 15. Trapp EG, Chisholm DJ, Freund J, Boutcher SH.

13.      Obes Rev. 2012 Oct;13(10):835-47 Thomas DM et al.

14.      US weight guidelines: is it also important to consider cardiorespiratory fitness? Int J Obes Relat Metab Disord. 1998 AugLee CD, Jackson AS, Blair SN.

15.      Alternate day fasting and endurance exercise combine to reduce body weight and favorably alter plasma lipids in obese humans. Obesity (Silver Spring). 2013 Feb 14.

16.      Hunter-Gatherer Energetics and Human Obesity. Herman Pontzer et al July 15 2012 PLOS.

17.      O'Keefe JH, Vogel R, Lavie CJ, Cordain L., Am J Med. 2010 Dec;123(12):1082-6. doi: 0.1016/j.amjmed.2010.04.026. Epub 2010 Sep 16.

18.      Six sessions of sprint interval training increases muscle oxidative potential and cycle endurance capacity in humans. J Appl Physiol (1985). 2005 Jun;98(6):1985-90. Epub 2005 Feb 10. Burgomaster KA, Hughes SC, Heigenhauser GJ, Bradwell SN, Gibala MJ.

19.      Short-term sprint interval versus traditional endurance training: similar initial adaptations in human skeletal muscle and exercise performance. J Physiol. 2006 Sep 15;575(Pt 3):901-11. Epub 2006 Jul 6. Gibala MJ, Little JP, van Essen M, Wilkin GP, Burgomaster KA, Safdar A, Raha S, Tarnopolsky MA.

20.     Physiological adaptations to low-volume, high-intensity interval training in health and disease. J Physiol. 2012 Mar 1;590(Pt 5):1077-84. doi: 10.1113/jphysiol.2011.224725. Epub 2012 Jan 30.   Gibala MJ, Little JP, Macdonald MJ, Hawley JA.

21.     The effects of high-intensity intermittent exercise training on fat loss and fasting insulin levels of young women.Int J Obes (Lond). 2008 Apr;32(4):684-91. doi: 10.1038/sj.ijo.0803781. Epub 2008 Jan 15. Trapp EG, Chisholm DJ, Freund J, Boutcher SH.

22.     The effect of high-intensity intermittent exercise on body composition of overweight young males. J Obes. 2012;2012:480467. doi: 10.1155/2012/480467. Epub 2012 Jun 6. Heydari M, Freund J, Boutcher SH.

23.     Macpherson RE, Hazell TJ, Olver TD, Paterson DH, Lemon PW. Med Sci Sports Exerc. 2011 Jan;43(1):115-22.

24.     Energy Intake of Obese Adolescents Is Spontaneously Reduced after Intensive Exercise: A Randomized Controlled Trial in Calorimetric Chambers. PLOS One  17 Jan 2012  The 24-h  Pascale Duché, Béatrice Morio.

25.     Aaron Sim, bit.ly/1aaGnvK International Journal of Obesity, online June 4, 2013.

26.     'Individual responses to combined endurance and strength training in older adults.' Karavirta L,  Med Sci Sports Exerc. 2011 Mar;43(3):484-90.

27.     JAMA. 2009 Apr 8;301(14):1439-50. doi: 10.1001/jama.2009.454. Efficacy and safety of exercise training in patients with chronic heart failure: HF-ACTION randomized controlled trial. O'Connor CM, Whellan DJ, Lee KL, Keteyian SJ, Cooper LS, Ellis SJ, Leifer ES, Kraus WE, Kitzman DW, Blumenthal JA, Rendall DS, Miller NH, Fleg JL,Schulman KA, McKelvie RS, Zannad F, Piña IL; HF-ACTION Investigators.

28.     Cardiovascular risk of high- versus moderate-intensity aerobic exercise in coronary heart disease patients published in Circulation in 2012

Sep 18;126(12):1436-40.

29.     High-intensity aerobic interval exercise in chronic heart failure.
Published in Circulation in 2012 Sep 18;126(12):1436-40. Curr Heart Fail
Rep. 2013 Jun;10(2):130-8. doi: 10.1007/s11897-013-0130-3. Meyer P,
Gayda M, Juneau M, Nigam A.

30.     When and Whom to Stretch: The Physician and Sportsmedicine -
Vol 33 - No. 3 - March 2005.

31.     Sports Medicine   Stretching and Injury Prevention June 2004,
Volume 34, Issue 7, pp 443-449  by Peter McNair.

32.     Warm-up reduces delayed onset muscle soreness but cool-
down does not: a randomised controlled trial, Australian J Physiotherapy
2007;53(2):91-5.

33.     "Towards the minimal amount of exercise for improving metabolic
health", Eur J Appl Physiol. 2012 Jul;112(7):2767-75. doi: 10.1007/s00421-
011-2254-z. Epub 2011 Nov 29. Metcalfe RS, Babraj JA, Fawkner SG,
Vollaard NB.

34.     Similar metabolic adaptations during exercise after low volume
sprint interval and traditional endurance training in humans. Burgomaster
KA, Howarth KR, Phillips SM, Rakobowchuk M, Macdonald MJ, McGee SL,
Gibala MJ, J Physiol. 2008 Jan 1;586(1):151 60. 8.

35.     "The Effects of high intensity intermittent exercise training
on fat loss and fasting insulin levels of young women" and J Obes.
2012;2012:480467. doi: 10.1155/2012/480467. Epub 2012 Jun 6. The effect
of high-intensity intermittent exercise on body composition of overweight
young males.

36.     Low- and high-volume of intensive endurance training
significantly improves maximal oxygen uptake after 10-weeks of training
in healthy men. PLoS One. 2013 May 29;8(5): e65382. Print 2013. Tjønna
AE, Leinan IM, Bartnes AT, Jenssen BM, Gibala MJ, Winett RA, Wisløff

U. Source K.G. Jebsen Center for Exercise in Medicine at Department of Circulation and Medical Imaging, Trondheim.

37.     High-intensity circuit training using body weight: maximum results with minimum effort  ACSM'S Health & Fitness Journal:  May/June 2013 - Volume 17 - Issue 3 - p 8–13.

38.     Appetite. 2005 Dec;45(3):272-8. Epub 2005 Sep 12.

39.     Chronobiology International; 2007; 24 (6) 1159-77.

40.      Ginger (Zingiber officinale) reduces muscle pain caused by eccentric exercise. J Pain. 2010 Sep;11(9):894-903. Black CD, Herring MP, Hurley DJ, O'Connor PJ.

41.     Breaking up prolonged sitting reduces postprandial glucose and insulin responses. Diabetes Care. 2012 May;35(5):976-83. doi: 10.2337/dc11-1931. Epub 2012 Feb 28. Dunstan DW, Kingwell BA, Larsen R, Healy GN, Cerin E, Hamilton MT, Shaw JE, Bertovic DA, Zimmet PZ, Salmon J, Owen N.

42.     Workman Publishing Company, US, 2004.

43.     The effects of free-living interval-walking training on glycemic control, body composition, and physical fitness in type 2 diabetic patients, Diabetes Care. 2013 Feb;36(2):228-36. doi: 10.2337/dc12-0658. Epub 2012 Sep 21.

44.     Effects of High-Intensity Interval Walking Training on Physical Fitness and Blood Pressure in Middle-Aged and Older People, Mayo Clin Proc. 2007 Jul;82(7):803-11., Nemoto K, Gen-no H, Masuki S, Okazaki K, Nose H.

# AUTHOR BIOGRAPHIES

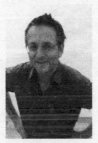

Michael Mosley did a first degree at Oxford University before training to be a doctor at the Royal Free Hospital in London. After qualifying he joined the BBC, where he has been a science journalist, executive producer and, more recently, a well-known television presenter. He has written and presented series on BBC One, Two, Three and Four as well as BBC Radio Four; and has won numerous television awards, including an RTS (Royal Television Award) and being named Medical Journalist of the Year by the British Medical Association. He is married to a doctor and has four children.

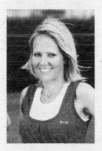

Peta Bee is an award-winning journalist who writes regularly for *The Times*, *Daily Mail* and *Sunday Times*. She has degrees in sports science and nutrition and is a qualified running coach. Peta won the Medical Journalists' Association's Freelance of the Year in 2008 and 2012 and appears regularly on television and radio. She has published several books on health and fitness and lives with her family in Berkshire.

# INDEX

# Acknowledgements

A big thanks to Toby MacDonald, Jenna Caldwell and Aidan Laverty for The Truth about Exercise and leading me to HIT.

To Mimi, Aurea and Rebecca for your friendship, editorial input and unwavering support

To Natalie, Andrew, Dan and Sophie – for making it happen.

Also many thanks to my GP, Sally Jenkins, who has always responded with great good humour to my outlandish requests; it's not easy being doctor to a self-experimenter.

*Michael Mosley*, Dec 2013